THE CHIROPRACTIC ALTERNATIVE

Published by J. P. TARCHER, INC.
Los Angeles

Distributed by HOUGHTON MIFFLIN CO.
Boston

The Chiropractic Alternative

A Spine Owner's Guide

Nathaniel Altman

Foreword by Mary Jane Newcomb, D.C., Ph.D.
Cleveland Chiropractic College

**Library of Congress Cataloging
in Publication Data**

Altman, Nathaniel, 1948–
The chiropractic alternative.

Bibliography: p. 197
Includes index.
1. Chiropractic—Popular works. I. Title.
RZ244.A38 615.5'34 79–93020
ISBN 0–87477–132–3

Library of Congress Catalog Card No.: 79–93020

Design by Barbara Monahan

Manufactured in the United States of America

Published by J. P. Tarcher, Inc.
9110 Sunset Blvd., Los Angeles, Calif. 90069

S 10 9 8 7 6 5 4 3 2 1
First Edition

This book is dedicated with gratitude to

CARL TOMPKINS, D.C.

DONALD M. EPSTEIN, D.C.

Contents

THE CHIROPRACTIC ALTERNATIVE

Foreword

For a reading public increasingly interested in natural methods of health and healing, no more appropriate outlook is conceivable than a book written by a layman who discovered chiropractic a few years ago as a result of a personal injury, returned for intermittent chiropractic care in the intervening years, and systematically conducted personal research in this field of health service.

Intrigued with the respect for human life inherent in chiropractic principles and already convinced that the body has the capacity to heal itself through an inborn intelligence, Nathaniel Altman, writer and lecturer, set out to study all areas of his subject. In *The Chiropractic Alternative*, he expresses his belief that chiropractic is here to stay and that, in fact, today's chiropractor is the doctor of the future.

The author provides background for us about the source of chiropractic and the scientific basis for its practice. He outlines the educational qualifications of the doctor of chiropractic for a public long holding the erroneous belief that the requirements for a chiropractic degree are meagre. He derives the definitive facts concerning the academic degree from a concentrated survey of catalogs, bulletins, and correspondence from each of the colleges and from responses received from national organizations related to the profession. In this book, Nathaniel

Altman offers insight into the ideal state of health, which the chiropractor attributes to a nervous system free from the pressure on nerves that results from misalignment of segments of the spinal column. Pointing out that health is the natural state of the body, Nat stresses the individual's seeking the foundation for "positive wellness."

During the period of his research, the writer determined not only to inform the lay person about chiropractic—the historical basis and the current status of the profession—but also to outline criteria for actually choosing a doctor in the field whose philosophy appears compatible with the person seeking care. Going beyond this careful advice, he takes the reader on a journey into a chiropractic office and describes a detailed procedure that should allay the apprehension of even the most cautious person in need of chiropractic health service.

The author of *The Chiropractic Alternative* is cognizant of the various philosophic tenets within the profession. He approaches objectively, but without passing judgment, the differences between the practitioner who treats the patient *by hand only* for the relief of symptoms and other manifestations of disease or trauma and the practitioner who takes a broad chiropractic outlook on patient care and who combines manipulative care and other therapeutic approaches. Over the years Nat has found that the scope of practice in chiropractic varies from office to office and from state to state. The evaluative and appreciative approach of the author embraces the various modes of practice in the profession, and his recognition of the importance of health maintenance through natural methods relates to the chiropractic field in toto.

Nat Altman has accomplished what a chiropractor could scarcely achieve. In the thirty-seven years since I entered chiropractic college, I have found that most people in the profession, regardless of method of health care delivery, tend to maintain a constant protective and defensive vigilance over a science and practice that is still in its infancy and still proving its worth to a medically oriented public. Such a stance makes objective value judgment from within difficult if not impossible. Nat has done both the difficult and the impossible.

Chiropractic is gaining in popularity and esteem both through the sheer number of people seeking the services of its practitioners and through the recognition by—and even support from—medical and other health-related organizations, accrediting bodies, and governmental agencies. The public is discovering that chiropractors are primary health care providers who refer patients to other doctors for consultation or service where need is indicated.

At the same time, chiropractic is steadily gaining in repute as a science supportable by fact. The profession recognizes that pure research in chiropractic must continue and that the outcomes must be carefully evaluated and adapted to the welfare of the public, and at no time in the history of chiropractic has there been such a body of research in progress as at present.

The Chiropractic Alternative is one of only a small collection of books published over the years that provides the public with an opportunity to know the advantages and the extent of chiropractic health care through the eyes of a nonchiropractor. The person who has never been a chiropractic patient may anticipate an adventure in natural health care through the reading of this book. One who has experienced chiropractic care should consider that the careful study along with a warmth of approach to the subject manifested here will assist in what Nat Altman has called "the educated decision" that all must make in the care and maintenance of health.

MARY JANE NEWCOMB, D.C., Ph.D.
Dean of Student Affairs
Cleveland Chiropractic College
Kansas City, Missouri

Preface

I first became aware of chiropractic when I tried to move my portable typewriter from a table to my desk. My back suddenly gave out as I lifted the typewriter and I doubled up in pain. Unable to sit in a chair, I spent the afternoon in bed, applying cold compresses and taking double doses of aspirin to reduce the pain.

Later that day a friend of mine convinced me to visit his chiropractor. The chiropractor led me to an adjusting table, had me lie down on my stomach, and with a careful thrust on my lower back made my spine "click" into place. Two thrusts later, I noticed that the pain was gone.

Five years later, I moved from New York to India, where the hot climate, the strange food, and the intense stress which came with my job took their toll. I began feeling very run down and was losing weight steadily. I was also suffering from an eye infection which I wasn't able to control with vitamins and medication.

I often met many visitors from abroad. One of these was a chiropractor from Australia. I decided to consult him. After a week of one gentle spinal adjustment and one acupressure treatment per day, my eye problem began to clear up and I had more energy than I felt in months. When the chiropractor finally left the city to continue his travels, over twenty grateful patients were on hand to bid him a sad farewell.

The following year, I injured my back while splitting logs in upstate New York. After I gave a talk on diet at a local senior citizens center, a member of the audience noticed my stiff walk and suggested that I visit her chiropractor, who helped relieve much of her arthritis. After two chiropractic adjustments, my back was better again.

This doctor also introduced me to chiropractic preventive health care, which involved more than treating symptoms when they arose. With regular chiropractic care my lower back problems (which were usually minor but chronic) disappeared and my hay fever symptoms the following spring were the mildest I had ever experienced.

Though I have had many positive experiences with chiropractic, I have found that others do not understand what it is really about. Organized medicine has condemned it as an unscientific cult which is useless and even dangerous. Others have touted it as a panacea for all human ills encompassing every therapy but drugs and surgery. It has been seen as a form of massage, a process featuring acupuncture and herbal remedies, a branch of medicine designed to stimulate nerves, a system confined to the treatment of bad backs and stiff necks, or a painful and dangerous procedure which cracks our bones and loosens our teeth.

In my growing enthusiasm, I looked for books to enlighten me. Most of the authors were chiropractors themselves. When not too difficult for the lay person to read, the books were often too simplistic and exaggerated. Other literature, such as one book published with the blessing of the American Medical Association, was little more than a propaganda tool of organized medicine. It attempted to isolate and eliminate chiropractic from the American health care mainstream.

Since there was a need for a carefully researched book for the lay person written by another lay person—a chiropractic patient—I decided to write *The Chiropractic Alternative*. As a writer and teacher of health subjects for over ten years, I wanted to use material from a variety of documented sources both within and outside the chiropractic profession. I felt the need to find out how the early pioneers of chiropractic viewed their young science and to investigate some of the controversies within the profession which are often avoided by chiropractic authors. My hope is that this book will provide you with the tools to make an educated decision about the kind of health care you want for yourself and your family.

Chiropractic is a science less than ninety years old, yet the principles on which it is based trace their roots to ancient Greece and the teachings of Hippocrates. In an age when people are questioning the extensive use of drugs and surgery in health care, one of the most outstanding qualities of chiropractic is its respect for the human body. Its primary goals are to regain and maintain good health, to restore normal transmission of nerve impulses, and to allow the body to heal itself through its inborn intelligence without stimulating or inhibiting functions. This is vital for resistance to disease and the healing process. In addition, it is effective, safe, and economical. For these reasons, millions of people have chosen the chiropractic alternative as their primary health care delivery system.

Acknowledgments

I would like to thank the following people, whose inspiration, editorial assistance, suggestions, criticism, and support were crucial to the successful completion of the manuscript: Mildred Aissen, Sadie Altman, Marjorie Bair, Amy Berkower, Julie Burger, M.T., Elissa DeWitt, Donald Epstein, D.C., Janice Gallagher, Albert Gani, Judith Gani, Mathilde Gasser, Eleanor Gilpatrick, Ph.D., Alan Hare, D.C., Thomas Kloiber, D.C., Amy Lebolt, Peter Massey, Bridget Mondello, Mary Jane Newcomb, D.C., Rose Oland, Jane Redicker, Michael Sherman, Laura Siegel, D.C., Patrick Sullivan, Carl Tompkins, D.C.

I would also like to gratefully acknowledge the help and/or permission to use material from the following corporations: The Foundation for Chiropractic Education and Research for permission to reproduce several anatomical drawings from *Chiropractic Health Care;* The International Chiropractors Association for generously supplying me with a wealth of reference material; Murdoch Engineering, Inc., for their photograph of the Thermeter; Williams Manufacturing for the photograph of their Zenith® Hylo™ adjusting table; and the Parker Chiropractic Research Foundation for their chart on the effects of spinal misalignments.

Introduction: What the Chiropractic Alternative Will Do for You

DURING THE SEVENTIES, AMERICA WITNESSED A groundswell of interest in alternative forms of health care. There is every indication the trend will continue well into the eighties and beyond. Chiropractic is one of these alternative ways to health, and in less than ninety years has become the largest drugless health system in the world. Discovered in the United States by Daniel David Palmer in 1895, chiropractic is now the second largest health care system in the United States, after traditional allopathic medicine.

Despite many years of desperate attempts by the American Medical Association and other groups to suppress its growth, over ten million Americans choose the chiropractic alternative every year. In addition to its growing popularity in the United States and Canada, chiropractic has spread all over the world.

Chiropractic is a unique health care science that deals with the vital relationship between the nervous system and the spinal column and with the role of this relationship in the restoration and maintenance of health. The philosophy of chiropractic teaches that our ability to adapt to changes in our internal and external environment is essential to the maintenance of life and health. An unobstructed flow of nerve impulses from the brain through the spinal nerves and onward to every body cell will help us achieve the balance, harmony and vitality we need to enjoy vibrant health and a long, productive life.

Contrary to popular belief, the scope of chiropractic extends far beyond the treatment of back pain and stiff necks. Chiropractic has been recognized for its ability to promote the total health and integration of the body because it focuses on the ability of the body to heal itself from the inside out. Chiropractic encourages us to take personal responsibility for our lives by teaching us to preserve our health rather than merely treating the symptoms of disease. It is in harmony with modern trends like healthy eating, exercise, body ecology and holistic health care. This effective and economical way to cope with America's health crisis offers great promise to those who suffer from ill health as well as those who want to stay healthy and active throughout their lives. Chiropractic cannot guarantee us a state of positive wellness—no health care system can. However, the goal of chiropractic is to help lay the foundation for positive wellness by keeping the nervous system free from impingements by spinal misalignments, which brings about a condition known in chiropractic as "dis-ease."

Bartlett Joshua Palmer, the son of the founder of chiropractic, was the first to teach that the term dis-ease does not imply "disease" as we know it, but rather a lack of harmony (or ease) within the human organism. He defined dis-ease as *that condition which allows illness (or disease) to exist:* it is *dis-order* and *mis-alignment*. According to Palmer, dis-eased bodies all have one thing in common: they are not working correctly and are malfunctioning in their areas of weakness.

Since its discovery in 1895, chiropractic has helped millions of people around the world to prevent dis-ease. They have found that chiropractic's preventive approach has helped keep them healthy at a reasonable cost. Some have found that chiropractic adjustments, greatly refined since 1895, have relieved painful back and neck problems including whiplash injuries, neuralgia, sciatica, bursitis, tendonitis, lumbago, disc problems, and muscle sprains. In addition, many have discovered that chiropractic has been successful in helping their bodies control organic disorders like hypertension, arthritis, rheumatism, bronchial asthma, allergies, nervous tension, chronic fatigue, heart trouble, and a host of other ailments, some of which did not respond well to medical therapy.

Chiropractic patients represent a wide variety of backgrounds and include preschool children, retired adults, Olympic athletes, factory workers, secretaries, teachers, dancers, farmers, mail carriers, truck drivers, firefighters, homemakers, and architects. Many outstanding Americans, including Eleanor Roosevelt, Bruce Jenner, Melvin Belli, Burt Reynolds, James Arness, and Rocky Marciano, have been among chiropractic's enthusiastic supporters.

This book will introduce you to the chiropractic alternative and how it can keep you well. The first part explains what chiropractic is, and how it works with your body's natural ability to heal itself from the inside out. You will learn what it can do for you, how long it takes to get well, and what happens when you visit a chiropractor. In addition, it will focus on the chiropractic profession itself, and explore modern chiropractic education and professional standards to help you select your personal chiropractor. Finally, the book will explore what chiropractors call "constructive survival values," offering practical guidance regarding stress management, diet, and exercise which you can follow to enhance the benefits of regular chiropractic care.

The chiropractic alternative is a unique health system.

Whether you are currently enjoying good health and want to maintain it, or are bothered by a problem which does not respond to conventional treatment, *The Chiropractic Alternative* is worth looking into. It will help you make an informed decision about the value of chiropractic care and will show you how to beat the high cost of health care today.

Part 1

SEEKING WELLNESS

1

The Evidence: Dramatic Results

A MIDDLE-AGED EXECUTIVE NEARLY GAVE UP his job because his migraine headaches were, as he said, "driving me up the wall." After six chiropractic adjustments, both the frequency and intensity of his headaches were sharply reduced.

A young woman had not had her period for three years. After four months of chiropractic care, she resumed her normal menstrual cycle.

A handyman sprained his back lifting machinery and could barely walk. Five minutes after a chiropractic adjustment, he was playfully lifting the chiropractor's child and tossing him into the air.

A teenage girl was taking six prescription drugs to control nine different allergies. After three weeks of chiropractic care, she was free of allergy symptoms and stopped taking drugs.

A 50-year-old man was told that he needed surgery to repair a herniated disc. After only two chiropractic adjustments, he returned to his amazed medical doctor who cancelled the operation.

An elderly woman dying of cancer received regular chiropractic care in place of narcotic drugs. Although she did not have a remission, she was able to live her last days with dignity.

If you walk into any chiropractor's office, the chances are good that patients will eagerly relate the "miracles" they have experienced thanks to chiropractic: "Chiropractic cured my back trouble." "It gave me sleep after years of insomnia and sleeping pills." "It lowered my blood pressure." "My arthritis is finally under control." "My child is no longer hyperkinetic and is doing well in school." "Chiropractic has relieved my constipation."

Before reviewing the evidence from over eighty years of clinical research, it is important to remember that chiropractic was not designed specifically to cure disease or directly treat symptoms, but to remove nerve interference. Chiropractic maintains that disturbances of the nervous system such as *subluxations* (a condition in which one or more vertebrae of the spine are out of alignment to the extent that a nerve is impinged and normal transmission of nerve energy is obstructed) can be the cause of aggravated dis-ease which may eventually lead to disease symptoms. Due to reflex action, almost any part of the nervous system may directly or indirectly cause sympathetic reactions in another part of the body. For example, a subluxation may trigger a headache, an asthmatic syndrome, or another nerve related problem, although it may not be the sole cause.

Since every tissue and organ of the body is connected and controlled by nerves from the spinal cord and brain, removal of nerve interference can bring dramatic results. With careful adjustments, the chiropractor releases our natural healing forces, which have the potential to relieve almost every ailment known.

Before considering medical evidence, we need to make a clear distinction between chiropractic *adjustments* and *manipulation*. An adjustment is the application of a rapid, sudden, and precise force (known in the profession as a "dynamic thrust") to a specific point of the vertebra *with the primary intention of allowing the body to remove nerve interference.* It is the body's reaction to the applied force which realigns structure as a secondary effect. A manipulation, on the other hand, is often a nonspecific, generalized procedure that resets bones, increases range of movement, and realigns joint structure with the intent to stimulate or inhibit body functions. For example, a practitioner who massages and then twists the neck and head in order to bring about a greater range of movement would be performing a manipulation.

Some chiropractors claim that since an adjustment is far more exacting than the average manipulation, it is often more effective in removing nerve interference. Though much of the following evidence is based on manipulation, remember that positive results from it can be equalled or surpassed by specific chiropractic adjustments.

Since the days of the founder, Daniel David Palmer, chiropractic has been exiled to the fringes of the health care mainstream by the organized medical profession. It has been denied the private and public funding that has gone toward medical research. As a result, most of the data concerning the effectiveness of this approach has been collected by chiropractors themselves. Even as organized medicine condemns it, however, traditional medical research offers an abundance of data that directly and indirectly attests to the value of chiropractic as a safe, effective means to help the patient overcome a wide variety of ailments.

BAD BACKS, STIFF NECKS, AND MORE: RELIEF FOR ORTHOPEDIC CASES

When most people think about chiropractors, they think of sore backs, stiff necks, and disc problems. These are the most common complaints among patients, but arthritis, rheumatism, sciatica, gout, postural deformities, muscle spasm, whiplash, nerve conditions, tennis elbow, and other kinds of sports injuries are also treated.

An article from the *British Medical Journal* entitled "Low Back Pain Treated by Manipulation" reported that 50 percent of the patients treated by spinal manipulation were free of symptoms by the end of one week. Only 27 percent of those receiving bed rest and drugs could claim similar results. Within three weeks, 87 percent of the manipulated patients were discharged from treatment, while only 60 percent of the others were.

A 1977 study of records from the Wisconsin Worker's Compensation Fund compared chiropractic with medical care in cases of industrial back injuries. The average compensation time for a chiropractic patient was 13.2 days at a cost of $145.64. A patient receiving medical care was compensated 18.3 days at an average cost of $267.58.

Investigative research has linked tennis elbow with a fixation of the cervical (neck) area of the spine. It also related rheumatoid arthritis to compression of the spinal nerves by bones and neck pain, sciatica, neuralgia, lumbago, and intercostal neuritis to misalignments of the spine.

Another common disorder caused by spinal nerve compression is *referred pain*, which is pain perceived by the brain as coming from a site other than its true origin. The *Journal of the American Medical Association* reported that a ruptured vertebral disc could produce a pain simulating angina. Research by Neville T. Ussher, M.D., found that spinal curvature resulting in nerve interference could produce radiating pain in different parts of the body with symptoms resembling gall bladder disease, appendicitis, gastritis, ulcer, colitis, spastic constipation, and other forms of irritation. The January 1948 issue of the *American Heart Journal* reported that nerve root pain in the midback can simulate, and is often mistaken for, coronary heart disease. Like a heart attack, the pain can radiate to the jaw, the upper left arm, and even cause a choking sensation in the throat. In some cases, spinal manipulation brought immediate relief.

The fact that chiropractic can correct the cause of many musculoskeletal disorders was underscored by the prestigious Commission of Inquiry into Chiropractic in New Zealand. It undertook the most complete and objective study of the science to date. Authorized by the Governor-General, the Commission heard testimony from hundreds of chiropractors and their patients, medical doctors, physiotherapists, and independent researchers from around the world. In its report, presented to the Parliament in Late 1979, the Commission stated: "There can be no doubt that chiropractic treatment is effective for musculoskeletal spinal disorders. As well as back pain, which makes up the great bulk of chiropractic practice, these must be taken to include migraine and pain radiating from the spine."

FROM THE HEAD DOWN: INSIDE-OUT HEALING

All major organs of the body are closely linked to the nervous system radiating from the spine. The wide variety of visceral disorders (involving the internal organs) that occur when spinal subluxations cause nerve interference should come as no surprise. Nevertheless, the list is impressive. Let's start from the head down.

An Australian study of migraine headaches at the University of New South Wales in Sydney compared chiropractic adjustments with manipulation by medical doctors and physiotherapists. Results showed that after two months, the chiropractic group showed a 40 percent reduction in frequency of attack and a 43 percent reduction in pain intensity. The others reported only 34 percent reduction in frequency of attack and 43 percent reduction in pain intensity. This study confirmed the results of an earlier study in Germany which attributed 80 percent of all headaches to vertebral subluxations. A Canadian study found that "at least 70 percent" of head pain arises from problems with the cervical spine and related structures.

Other research has shown that whiplash injury can damage nerves affecting the ear as well as cause recurring dizziness. Excessive motion of a cervical vertebrae also caused dizziness and blurred vision. An article in the British medical journal *Lancet* linked vertigo to subluxations in the neck. Irritation of the cervical nerves were related to nausea, headache, transitory deafness, blurred vision, and loss of balance. In the 1970 *Yearbook of the Academy of Applied Osteopathy*, a series of manipulative techniques for the treatment of eye conditions such as retinitis, conjunctivitis, early cataract, and glaucoma were included.

Moving down from the head, we find the *Journal of the American Medical Association* cited a possible relationship between hyperparathyroidism and spinal curvature. The *Journal of the American Osteopathic Association* found that 88 percent of subjects with cervical lesions also suffered from thyroid dysfunctions compared to 34 percent of thyroid dysfunction among subjects without cervical disturbance.

The *Annals of Allergy* explains that spinal curvature, which is correctable by manipulation, may interfere with the central nervous system and aggravate asthma. The *Journal of the American Osteopathic Association* discusses the beneficial uses of manipulation for the midback as an adjunct to diet and breathing exercises for asthmatics. Other medical references draw attention to its ability to lower blood pressure, fight against chronic lung disease, and improve the body's use of oxygen.

An article in a European medical journal described a case study on 100 ulcer patients and found that 86 percent suffered from spinal curvatures of some kind, and 90 percent showed pathological changes in the intervertebral discs. A 1967 report by the renowned Mayo Clinic related both urinary retention and incontinence to misaligned discs in the lower back.

Problems related to the sex organs have also been linked to spinal misalignments. The German journal *Manuelle Medezin* presented several arguments in favor of spinal manipulation for a variety of female disorders before and after giving birth. An article in the *Archives of Physical Medicine and Rehabilitation* and a letter in the *Journal of the American Medical Association* explain the physiological relationship between male sexual dysfunction and misalignments of the lower back.

WHAT ABOUT CANCER?

John C. has cancer, but after four months of chiropractic care he is in remission. Does that mean chiropractic cures cancer? A responsible chiropractor would answer in the negative, but proceed to ask a more important question: Can a physiologically sound organism, freed from dis-ease and nerve interference, fight cancer? The answer to *this* is yes. According to Gardner's *Fundamentals of Neurology*, autonomic functions of the nervous system (such as resistance to disease) are affected by spinal trauma. When nerve interference is removed, normal nerve activity can return. Then, major body functions like immunity to bacteria and virus can function at optimum level to fight a threat like cancer cells. An article in *Time* magazine included the following comments regarding this important issue:

> Sir Frank MacFarlane Burnet, an Australian, and Dr. Lewis Thomas, who has just been appointed President of Memorial Sloane-Kettering Cancer Center, suggested a relationship between the immune system and cancerous growth. They postulated that in addition to protecting the

> body from invaders, the immune system has the duty to police cell growth and prevent the survival and reproduction of abnormal or "outlaw" cells.

Burrows' *Textbook of Microbiology* agrees: "Cases of spontaneous regression of human tumors suggest that an active immunological response may be holding the growth in check."

Responsible chiropractors will never promise that they can cure cancer although Dr. Tedd Koren, a chiropractor from Pennsylvania, believes that chiropractic is beneficial whether or not the cancer patient is under the care of a medical doctor. In the *International Review of Chiropractic*, Koren points out that cancer is the result of a body not working correctly for many years. Removing nerve interference by chiropractic adjustments may help a body which works improperly to work properly. It has a better chance of fighting off cancer. For those under medical care, Dr. Koren feels an uninterrupted nerve supply will give the patient greater natural resistance, thereby avoiding iatrogenic disease, a consequence of cancer therapy.

WHAT CHIROPRACTIC LITERATURE SAYS

In the preceding pages we cited a small part of the extensive medical literature concerning ailments which respond to spinal manipulation and chiropractic adjustments. Although some critics feel chiropractic literature is less objective than data from other sources, the following may help us understand why so many feel it has brought hope when medical science was unable to help them.

A partial listing of cases successfully treated at Spears Chiropractic Hospital includes incapacitating headaches, triple vision and blackouts, convulsions, disability due to stroke, rheumatoid arthritis, cerebral palsy, muscular dystrophy, hyperthyroidism, goiter, emphysema, bronchitis, and several skin disorders including scleroderma (thickening of the skin) and vascular dermatitis. Other clinics have reported similar success with a variety of visceral disorders. Dr. Lyle W. Sherman saw dramatic results while he was head of the Palmer Chiropractic Clinic in Davenport. According to Sherman, some of the ailments which responded to chiropractic care included cirrhosis and cancer of the liver, epilepsy, encephalitis, hydrocephalus, tumors, and multiple sclerosis.

However, the most impressive reports on chiropractic's success with paralysis were published in *The Chiropractic Story* by Marcus Bach, Ph.D. Winifred Gardella, the 1955 March of Dimes poster girl, underwent two-and-a-half years of unsuccessful medical treatment to restore her lifeless arms and legs. A chiropractor heard of her case. After six months of chiropractic adjustments, she put her crutches aside and walked. Another dramatic case involved 11-year-old Donny Spackman of suburban Chicago. Confined to a wheelchair with paralysis, after just ten days of chiropractic care, he got out of his wheelchair and walked.

The New Zealand Commission of Inquiry into Chiropractic heard many cases similar to these but was unable to conclude that chiropractic care would guarantee such positive results all the time. After reviewing hundreds of cases, the Commission prepared the following, carefully worded statement:

> On the question whether spinal manual therapy (chiropractic adjustments) can influence organic and/or visceral disorders, the Commission is satisfied that in some cases this is at least a possibility. Moreover, there is enough anecdotal material to satisfy the Commission that in some instances chiropractors have been able to relieve disorders of this nature which seem to have defeated orthodox medicine. . . . Without [the chiropractor], the quality of

life of many would be less bearable. Their pain and frustration are undoubtedly relieved.

THE CASE FOR PSYCHOLOGICAL WELL-BEING

It is well known that a healthy nervous system is basic to good mental health. Nerve impairments can produce localized stress or psychological syndromes like depression or hyperactivity. A recent study of delinquent children, undertaken at Yale University, found that 98.6 percent of the more violent youths had at least one sign of neurological impairment as opposed to 66.7 percent of the less violent group.

Although extensive comparative research still needs to be done, pilot studies have indicated that regular chiropractic care can have a dramatic effect on people with severe emotional problems. The Psychoeducational and Guidance Services in Texas compared traditional methods of treatment with chiropractic. It was carried out during the school year of 1973–1974 with 24 children who showed marked behavioral and learning problems due to neurological dysfunction. By the end of the study, the results showed that spinal adjustments produced marked improvement with none of the adverse effects caused by drugs.

Another pilot study sponsored by the National Committee on Psychology of the American Chiropractic Association in 1947 did the same comparison with a group of 350 children and adults, 114 of whom were institutionalized. It was performed by George W. Hartmann, Ph.D., and Herman Schwartz, D.C. All the patients were evaluated before the testing began. Seventy-five percent of those who had undergone medical and psychiatric therapy showed "no change" in their progress. Only 13 percent reported some improvement. Ten percent (or 27) reported that their progress had deteriorated.

After receiving regular chiropractic adjustments, however, an impressive 81 percent of the patients were found to have experienced a marked improvement. Four percent (or 13) of the participants showed no improvement. Only six patients (1.5 percent of the total) were found to be worse than before treatment started. Approximately 42 percent of the patients received no psychotherapy while under chiropractic care. Only 8.5 percent received in-depth psychiatric counseling during the course of the investigation.

The findings of the Hartmann/Schwartz study are impressive and a seven-year follow-up substantiated the lasting benefits of chiropractic care. However, it should not be seen as a panacea for emotional problems, because factors such as childhood conditioning, diet, and environment all play a role in mental health.

Anxiety, hyperactivity, and tension have reached epidemic proportions in this country. The major "pseudo-solution" has been the use of many dangerous drugs, and we can no longer ignore the potential of chiropractic as an alternative. It works to maintain the integrity of the nervous system, which in turn helps us adapt better to daily stress. It can be an effective form of preventive mental health care. In addition, the possibility of chiropractic being used in conjunction with therapeutic approaches, such as analysis, bioenergetics, meditation, and Gestalt, can offer new possibilities for the prevention and treatment of emotional problems.

CHIROPRACTIC AND THE ATHLETE

Chiropractic has been of tremendous benefit for thousands of athletes everywhere. It is used preventively to avoid injury, to help the athlete keep in top health, or as a simple, effective form of treating injuries. Rocky Marciano, Bruce Jenner, and Roberto Clemente are among its devoted fans.

Dr. Leroy Perry from Pasadena, California, drew national attention to his work with Olympic and professional athletes. According to a recent article in *Sports Illustrated,* his patients have included Olympic team members like gold-medal runner Alberto Juantorena of Cuba, high jumper Dwight Stones, long jumper Arnie Robinson, discuse thrower Jan Svendsen, skier Suzy Chaffee, javelin thrower Kate Schmidt, and professional athletes such as football players Alex Karras and Ricky Bell and baseball players Rick Monday, Don Sutton, and Jim Palmer.

Although the Sports Medicine Council deterred Perry and other chiropractors from adjusting Olympic athletes during trials, the U.S. Olympic Committee's Advisory Council voted unanimously to include chiropractors on all of the teams. Dr. David Martin, exercise physiologist and Associate Professor at Georgia State University, explains: "From the point of view of the athletes, Dr. Perry has made fantastic progress in both healing and prevention."

CHIROPRACTIC AND THE OLDER ADULT

Chiropractic's preventive approach to health has been of great benefit to athletes. However, many people of retirement age have also discovered that regular chiropractic care keeps them active and healthy in their later years. Once, I presented a talk to a senior citizen's group. Afterwards, several members of the audience told me about dramatic benefits they experienced with a local chiropractor (whom I later consulted for my own chiropractic care). "Dr. Carl helped my arthritis." "Chiropractic helped reduce my blood pressure and my medical doctor took me off medication." "Before I found chiropractic I had to use a cane because of my sciatica." These comments are typical of older adults who turned to chiropractic as an adjunct or alternative to traditional medical care.

Chiropractic care is especially important for seniors. As a person ages, muscles which maintain normal alignment of the spine lose their tone. The vertebrae tend to become misaligned, affecting spinal nerves which lead to the major organs, joints, and tissues of the body. Serious problems such as arthritis, hypertension, constipation, and other digestive disorders may result from nerve interference and dis-ease.

This method of health care is gaining popularity among older adults. It is painless, both corrective and preventive, and is reasonably priced. Regular chiropractic adjustments insure an uninterrupted nerve supply to keep every part of the body functioning at optimal level for the longest possible time. It can make youthfulness a question of vibrant health rather than of one's physical age.

CHIROPRACTIC FOR BABIES AND CHILDREN

Already used by older adults, chiropractic is becoming even more popular with their grandchildren. Since the spine is subject to frequent strain from birth through a child's accident-prone formative years, a growing number of parents are making sure their children receive chiropractic care as early as possible.

The Birth Trauma: The First Subluxation

Perhaps the most serious cause of early subluxation is the current birthing process. Earlier methods utilized midwives and birthing stools. Today, hospital births are easier on the doctor but harder on the baby. He pulls, stretches, and twists the infant's body, following this with a hard slap on the baby's rump. The seriousness of spinal injuries at birth has been ignored until recently. Dr. Abraham Towbin, affiliated with

Harvard University Medical School, reported that spinal cord and brain stem injury is present in up to 33 percent of newborn deaths. This translates as 20,000 infant fatalities a year in this country alone. Dr. Towbin wrote:

> Mechanical stress imposed by obstetrical manipulation—even the application of standard orthodox procedures—may prove intolerable to the fetus. . . . Forceful longitudinal traction during delivery, particularly when combined with flexion and torsion of the vertebral axis, is thought to be the most important cause of neonatal spinal injury.

Most children do not die at birth from such injuries, although some chiropractors speculate they may be a factor in Sudden Infant Death Syndrome (SIDS) or other life-threatening conditions during the first year. A case in point involved Edward G., of Dixon, Illinois, in September 1942. He suffered a severe asthmatic attack with respiratory failure at eight months of age. Since no medical doctor was available, his mother summoned a local chiropractor, who happened to be blind. She related the dramatic incident years later.

> Around 6 A.M. Eddie turned blue, his breath stopped right below the breastbone. I had heard about this blind chiropractor, Dr. Bend, and called him. He and his assistant came right away. After feeling around his body he said: "I cannot treat a baby that small. I might kill him and would it not be grist for the medicals if the baby should die under my hands?" Ed could hardly breathe and I begged him to try, assuring him that he would surely die soon anyway. His assistant pleaded also, so he held Ed up toward his shoulder, holding the baby's head in his right hand, and twisted it. I heard a click and gradually Ed started breathing better. Dr. Bend's head was drenched in perspiration

> while he kept Eddie's head firmly in the same position for a half an hour.
>
> He explained that the little bone in the spine that got out of place was no bigger (in a baby less than a year old) than an old fashioned pinhead and that it was a matter of time until nature would make this bone stay put. . . . I am grateful to him as long as I live.

At the time of this writing, Edward G. just celebrated his 39th birthday and has not suffered an asthma attack in 38 years.

Although not as dramatic as the case above, thousands of newborn babies may suffer from a variety of persistent nerve defects in their early years due to spinal injury and misalignment. Paralysis, muscle imbalance leading to poor coordination, respiratory problems, symptoms of cerebral palsy, mental retardation, epilepsy, cardiac arrhythmia, and a host of subtle nervous disorders may be present, yet undetected. For this reason, chiropractors suggest babies and small children receive spinal examinations as early as possible in order to detect subluxations and other problems.

As children grow older, they advise a regular program of preventive examination and spinal care. If your children are active (and most are) they will absorb more than their share of falls, jolts, jars, sprains, and strains in the home and outdoors. Often, these mishaps cause spinal pressure on sensitive nerves, setting the stage for serious problems later. Most subluxations are corrected through the normal movement of the spine, but serious misalignments call for the services of an expert. A chiropractor is specially trained to determine if your child has any of these problems. He is the only practitioner qualified to correct them with safe and effective chiropractic adjustments.

Proven to be safe and effective for children, its success with senior citizens, also, shows we are never too old to enjoy the benefits of chiropractic care. Its primary goal is prevention of dis-ease, but specific chiropractic adjustments affecting the nervous system directly, have indirectly helped millions cure themselves of ailments not responding to traditional medical therapy.

Despite growing popularity, most are not aware of chiropractic's long, turbulent history: its ancient roots, its difficult period of growth in America, and the relentless efforts to destroy the fledgling profession by organized medicine. In the following chapter we will examine the controversial history of chiropractic from its beginnings to its current status as the second largest health care delivery system in the West today.

2

Chiropractic: A Controversial History

CHIROPRACTIC WAS DISCOVERED LESS THAN A century ago, but its roots extend back to the beginnings of recorded history. One historian cites an ancient Kong Fou document from China, written about 2700 B.C., which describes tissue manipulation. An early Greek papyrus dating back to 1500 B.C. gives instructions on maneuvering the lower extremities to treat low back conditions. Manipulation of sprained, dislocated, displaced, and crushed vertebrae was used in early Egypt. A rare, surviving work, now called the *Edwin Smith Surgical Papyrus*, was studied by physicians some 1700 years before Christ. The following advice helped them make a proper diagnosis:

> If thou examinest [a man having] a sprain in a vertebra of his spinal column, thou shouldst say to him: "Extend now thy two legs [and] contract them both [again]." When he extends them both he contracts them both immediately because of the pain he causes in the vertebra of his spinal column in which he suffers.

Most of us would laugh at this test for something as obvious as back sprain, but early Egyptians may have actually discovered the complex relationship between the vertebrae, the spinal nerves, and the leg muscles.

"Foot walking" was a popular form of treatment for disease and other ailments in early Polynesia, and children used to walk along the backs of their ailing elders. Even today, ancient backwalking techniques are practiced by the Maori peoples of New Zealand.

Spinal manipulation was not limited only to the East. It was practiced in one form or another by the Sioux, Winnebago, and Creek peoples in North America. The Incas of South America used it for illness and back pain as did the Aztec, Toltec, Tarascan, Zoltec, and Mayan cultures of Mexico and Central America.

The greatest breakthrough took place in ancient Greece. The Father of Medicine, Hippocrates (460–357 B.C.), was the first physician to link spinal misalignments with ill health. His students were advised to "get knowledge of the spine, for this is the requisite for many diseases." They were taught the value and practice of special techniques described in several now-famous medical texts.

Hippocrates also designed the first table for making spinal adjustments. Fitted with various pulleys and clamps, his invention enabled the physician to make effective adjustments with a minimum of risk to the patient. A wooden wedge helped reduce spinal humps.

Other early physicians echoed Hippocrates' advice, but Claudius Galen (131–200 A.D.) stands out among them. A Greek physician who dominated medicine during the early Roman Empire, Galen was among the first to recognize the importance of the nervous system. As a result of his animal dissections (the dissection of humans was considered sinful), he discovered seven of the twelve important cranial nerves. The cervical, lumbar, and dorsal (thoracic) regions of the spine were also named and defined. Although understanding *human* anatomy took centuries, much of Galen's work had positive impact on the development of medicine.

The fall of the Roman Empire in 476 A.D. plunged twenty centuries of accumulated human knowledge into darkness. Hundreds of libraries were plundered and thousands of scientific documents were burned by invaders. The evolution of medicine was severely curtailed during this period appropriately known as the Dark Ages. Scientific inquiry and understanding were replaced with fear and superstition. The development of spinal manipulation was also set back during this time. The popping sound so commonly heard during treatment was thought to come from demons (then accepted as the cause of disease) which were being driven from the patient.

Despite this belief, the art of spinal manipulation was not lost completely. It was kept alive (often in secret) by mainly unschooled physicians throughout Europe, especially in the area known today as Germany.

By the Middle Ages, spinal manipulation became known to the public again, and it enjoyed wide popularity throughout the Renaissance when it was known as *bonesetting*. Using knowledge handed down from parent to child, early bonesetters were regarded as gifted healers who could treat a wide variety of illnesses, aches, and pains by manipulating bones into place again. Often successful when other treatment failed, it quickly spread throughout Europe and by the eighteenth century was one of the most recognized healing arts on the Continent.

Bonesetting didn't become popular in the United States until the following century, when it expanded with Western migration. One of the most famous practitioners in this country was Steven Sweet of Sag Harbor, Long Island, the head of a famous family of bonesetters. Though he was totally untrained and lacked a basic education, he treated many ailments that were beyond the ability of even highly trained medical doctors.

Interest in this skill wasn't limited to "uneducated" men like Steven Sweet. The renowned British surgeon Sir James Paget wrote an article entitled "Cases That Bonesetters Cure" for the January 5, 1865, issue of the *British Medical Journal*.

Dr. Wharton Hood of London shared his observations in the treatise *On Bonesetting*, which received wide acclaim in medical circles. "I was astounded," he wrote, "and often no less mortified, at the number and variety of instances in which the manipulators I have endeavoured to describe were followed by almost immediate cure." This success led to a greater interest in the spine among medical doctors, and several scholarly works were written during the nineteenth century as a result.

THE FIRST ADJUSTMENT: DOC! DOC! I HEAR!

It was September 18, 1895, in the middle of a busy work week in Davenport, Iowa. Harvey Lillard, janitor at the Putnam Building, was relating to Daniel David Palmer how he had become virtually deaf. Palmer was a magnetic healer (one that heals by laying on of hands) who practiced there. He later described the event in the book, *The Science, Art and Philosophy of Chiropractic*.

> Harvey Lillard, a janitor in the Ryan Block, where I had my office, had been so deaf for 17 years that he could not hear the racket of a wagon on the street or the ticking of a watch. I made inquiry as to the cause of his deafness and was informed that when he was exerting himself in a cramped, stooped position, he felt something give way in his back and immediately became deaf. An examination showed a vertebra racked from its normal position. I reasoned that if that vertebra was replaced, the man's hearing should be restored. With this object in view, a half-hour's talk persuaded Mr. Lillard to allow me to replace it. I racked it into position by using the spinous process as a lever and soon the man could hear as before.

After three adjustments in as many days, Lillard jumped up and cried "Doc! Doc! I hear!" For the first time in seventeen years, Harvey Lillard could make out the rumble of the horsedrawn trolleys four stories below. This was the birth of the science of chiropractic.

D. D. PALMER: THE FOUNDER (1845–1913)

As a boy, Daniel David Palmer would often take to the woods in search of skeletons of animals which had died the winter before. Sometimes along with them he brought home a small animal with a broken bone. He would apply tiny splints fashioned of twigs and strips of cloth; the bones always mended. His mother would say that young Daniel had "healing hands." Whenever a member of the family was ill, they would look to him for comfort. His interest in health continued into adolescence, when Daniel spent much of his free time reading books on anatomy and how the body worked.

After experience as a prosperous beekeeper and then as a fish peddler and grocer, he eventually settled in the small town of Letts, Iowa, a few miles from the Mississippi River.

At this point, Palmer resumed his reading and gradually became open to new ideas in health and metaphysics. He began to teach classes in business and lecture from town to town on the subject of phrenology, an ancient system of character analysis based on study of the shape and features of the skull. During a tour he met Paul Caster, an internationally known magnetic healer from nearby Burlington, Iowa. Visiting him several days later, Palmer was astounded by the collection of abandoned crutches, canes, and braces hanging on the office walls and soon became a student of Caster. Eventually he began his own practice in Burlington after rediscovering his early talents and interest in helping the sick.

Throughout nine years as a magnetic healer, Palmer read dozens of books on anatomy and physiology, devoting much time to the human spine. He learned the body receives nerve energy through the vertebral column. An impingement of the spinal nerves could inhibit the energy flowing from the brain through the nerves to various organs of the body. He concluded that misaligned vertebrae could well be a cause of disease.

With increasing success as a healer, Palmer shortened his name to "D. D." and began calling himself "Doctor," a rather common practice in those days. His knowledge of anatomy surpassed that of most doctors. Medical schools in those days required less than a year of attendance, and many of their graduates became itinerant practitioners who sold snake oil and other remedies of dubious value.

After D. D. Palmer made the dramatic discovery of chiropractic in 1895, he began to refine the technique and develop the philosophy for a new healing art. He wrote:

> The human body represents the actions of three laws, spiritual, mechanical and chemical, united as one. . . . As long as there is perfect union of these three there is health. This machine, like all others, is run by power, called mental impulses, made in the brain and connected with the body by a system of nerves thru [sic] which this force passes in currents, including the higher exemplification of intellectual power. Functions are names given to these actions, any interference to the passage of these vitalizing currents produces abnormal functions—disease.

One of Palmer's most devoted patients was Rev. Samuel H. Weed, who had been successfully treated for sciatica. Rev. Weed coined the term *chiropractic* from the Greek words χιερ, "hand" and πρακτοσ, "done." In Palmer's words, the term *chiropractor* is "a hand practitioner—one who repairs or one who adjusts."

In 1897, D. D. Palmer established the Palmer Infirmary and Chiropractic School in Davenport, Iowa. Featuring a three-month course, the new institution attracted a diversity of students including several women, medical doctors, osteopaths, and surgeons. Among them was Dr. Alfred F. Walton of the Medical College of the University of Pennsylvania, who had graduated from Harvard University Medical School. After becoming a chiropractor, he lectured and wrote extensively in support of the new profession, helping to make it respectable in the eyes of many physicians.

B. J. PALMER: THE DEVELOPER (1881–1961)

Bartlett Joshua Palmer is hailed as the second most important figure in the history of chiropractic. Fourteen years old when the new science was discovered, he helped elevate it to the second largest health care system in America by the time he died in 1961. During his lifetime he was a brilliant and colorful chiropractor, writer, teacher, lecturer, and radio pioneer. He saved chiropractic from extinction in its early years and preserved many of the original principles laid down by his father. Bart was in Palmer School's first graduating class in 1902. He eventually joined his father as co-administrator.

In 1906, they had the first taste of organized medicine's opposition to chiropractic. Although D. D. Palmer had enjoyed the friendship and respect of many medical doctors, osteopaths, and homeopaths for over ten years, both he and B. J. were arrested for practicing medicine without a license.

Within a year of this incident, Daniel David sold his share to his son and left Davenport to set up chiropractic schools in Oklahoma and Oregon. Eventually he began a monumental 1008-page text, *The Science, Art and Philosophy of Chiropractic*, and settled in Los Angeles, where he lived in relative obscurity until his death in 1913.

Back in Davenport, B. J. renamed his school the Palmer School of Chiropractic and moved it to the present campus. It was later known as the "Chiropractic Fountain Head," and the majority of the world's chiropractors have graduated from there. By the end of 1906, B. J. Palmer had published the first major textbook on chiropractic. He married Mabel Heath, an early student at PSC, who had also studied anatomy at Rush Medical College in Chicago. Known as the "First Lady of Chiropractic," she wrote a widely respected book on anatomy, served on the faculty of the Palmer School, and played a leading role in attracting women to the profession until her death in 1949.

B. J. was embroiled in controversy for much of his life. As a man of determination who was strict in philosophy, he incurred the wrath of many chiropractors who did not want to limit chiropractic to manual spinal adjustments. Then he alienated a group of his own students and faculty in 1909 by introducing the *spinograph*, the first X-ray machine ever used to detect spinal misalignments. They objected to the use of anything but hands in chiropractic analysis (Palmer felt that while chiropractic *adjustments* should be limited to hands only, chiropractic *analysis* need not). Leaving the Palmer School during one of B. J.'s classes, the group established the Universal Chiropractic College several blocks down the street. Ironically enough, the UCC began using the spinograph later. After the college moved to Pittsburgh in 1918, its researchers invented the first X-ray machine that photographed the entire spine while the patient stood upright. This was very important. Spinographs could show, for the first time, the effects of unequal leg length, pelvic distortion, and body stress under the normal influence of gravity.

Fifteen years later, Palmer's introduction of the *neurocalometer* sparked another exodus of faculty and students. It was a hand held device featuring two heat-sensitive prongs designed to measure temperature differences on either side of the spine without causing pain to the patient. Since they can indicate the existence of nerve interference, the neurocalometer and similar devices are widely used today to locate subluxations throughout the vertebral column.

After the death of D. D. Palmer in 1913, chiropractic began to experience rapid growth. Kansas and North Dakota became the first states to legalize it. Half of the 48 states had recognized chiropractic by 1920, followed by the Canadian province of Ontario. Dozens of colleges sprang up across the country. Two national organizations were established to represent the growing profession: The National (now American) Chiropractic Association and the Universal (now International) Chiropractors Association, which was founded by B. J. Palmer himself.

In addition to B. J. Palmer, other outstanding chiropractors played an important role. Dr. John J. Nugent urged chiropractic colleges to raise their educational standards, and his efforts helped bring the profession closer to serious consideration by established academic accrediting agencies. Dr. Willard Carver once presided over four colleges at the same time. He extended D. D. Palmer's original concepts to include soft tissue manipulation and a form of positive thinking he called "mental science." Dr. Leo J. Spears founded the Spears Chiropractic Hospital and Sanitarium in Denver,* now the world's largest hospital for intensive chiropractic care. Dr. L. M. Rogers, President of the National Chiropractic Association, encouraged chiropractors to be more scientific in their approach.

ORGANIZED MEDICINE: THE ENEMY

Expansion of the new approach into primary health care alarmed the organized medical profession. The American Medical Association's first tactic was to try and isolate it. In 1933, the Judicial Council of the AMA discouraged members from

*927 Jersey, Denver, CO 80220

consulting with chiropractors or referring patients to them for help: "The physician who maintains professional relations with cult practitioners would seem to exhibit a lack of faith in the correctness and efficacy of scientific medicine and to admit that there is merit to cult practitioners."

Another tactic was to require chiropractic students to take the Basic Science Exam which was designed for medical doctors and osteopaths. B. J. Palmer loudly condemned it and claimed that since chiropractic was neither medicine nor a form of medical therapy, students should not have to take an examination designed for the medical profession. Nevertheless, by the 1930s the exam was commonplace, nearly ruining the chiropractic profession in America. Between 1927 and 1944 only 28 percent of the students passed and many chiropractic schools were forced to close their doors.

After B. J. Palmer's death in 1961, organized medicine was more determined than ever to send chiropractic to destruction. The earlier 1933 AMA statement was changed to a firm command. Any medical doctor who associated with a chiropractor was branded as "unethical." In 1963, the Board of Trustees established a "Committee on Quackery" to contain and eliminate the profession. A confidential memorandum to the AMA Department of Investigation dated September 21, 1967, revealed the Committee's short-range goals:

1. Doing everything within our power to see that chiropractic coverage under Title 18 of the Medicare Law is not obtained.
2. Doing everything within our power to see that recognition of listing by the U.S. Office of Education of a chiropractic accrediting agency is not achieved.
3. To encourage continued separation of the two national chiropractic organizations.
4. To encourage state medical societies to take the initiative in their state legislatures in regard to legislation that might affect the practice of chiropractic.

The long range goal was that "chiropractic licensure should be made so difficult that eventually more chiropractors are dying than new chiropractic licenses are granted." Radiologists were told that providing X-ray services to chiropractors and their patients was unethical. The Radiological Society of New York warned, "A practicing radiologist in the State of New York shall have no voluntary association with cultists of chiropractic, including consultation and the acceptance of referrals." High schools were not exempt from the conspiracy. A letter from the President of the Pennsylvania Medical Society to guidance counselors condemned the new health method as an "unscientific cult" adding, "To direct a highly motivated and intelligent student into a career in chiropractic would indeed be a loss to society."

CHIROPRACTIC FIGHTS BACK—AND WINS

Despite efforts to assure itself of a health care monopoly in the United States and to deny freedom of choice to American consumers, the AMA was unable to eliminate or even contain chiropractic. In 1974, four historical events took place which were major victories:

1. Louisiana became the last of fifty states to grant a separate board of licensure.
2. The Office of Education of the Department of Health, Education and Welfare authorized the Council of Chiropractic Education (CCE) to begin accrediting training colleges.
3. Congress included chiropractic in its Medicare program.
4. Congress authorized a $2 million study on the scientific basis of chiropractic, which resulted in a landmark 1975 congress on The Research Status of Spinal Manipula-

tive Therapy. This gave practitioners equal status with other health care professionals.

Today, almost every community in the nation is served by a doctor of chiropractic. Enrollment in training colleges is at an all time high. Because education costs are less than in traditional medicine, five new schools have opened since 1970 to accommodate students. More than 600 insurance companies provide for chiropractic care in health and accident policies. Claims are honored under Worker's Compensation programs in the U.S. and Canada. Millions of union members and many national employee organizations are eligible for care.

Chiropractic is here to stay. In fact, the American Medical Association has recently revised its earlier prohibition against medical doctors associating with chiropractors: "A physician may refer a patient for diagnosis or therapeutic services to another physician, a limited practitioner, or any other provider of health care services permitted by law to furnish such services, whenever he believes that this may benefit the patient."

Is the battle over? Not quite. Despite several antitrust suits against the AMA and related organizations (one suit was instituted by the New York State Attorney General in 1979), organized medicine can be expected to continue its opposition. Many chiropractors fear the next phase of the struggle will be chiropractic's gradual absorption into medical therapy as was the osteopathic profession. The controversy will be closely watched by chiropractors and patients alike, for it will determine the type of health care we and our children will receive in the years to come.

3

Chiropractic: What It Really Is

NEARLY EVERYONE HAS HEARD OF CHIROPRACTIC. Over ten million Americans used it in 1980, yet were still unfamiliar with the theory behind it. Some feel that chiropractic is basically intended for treating stiff necks and sore backs only. Others believe it can cure any disease known to humanity, even cancer. Still others have trouble distinguishing the approach from traditional medical therapy except that medical doctors use drugs and surgery and chiropractors do not. It is also confused with health systems like osteopathy, acupressure, and massage.

The purpose of this chapter is to clear up the trouble. With the help of original material taken from the writings of D. D. Palmer and others, we will explore why chiropractic is a distinct healing art.

In 1890, it was well known that the central nervous system—brain, spinal cord, and nerves—controlled the entire body. The brain generates energy. The energy is directed down the spinal cord in the form of electrical impulses or messages. The impulses leave the spine at various points between the vertebrae to travel along nerve pathways to organs and tissues where they guide every function.

There is a return cycle as well. Each part of the body is constantly sending messages regarding its function and environment to the brain. This information is processed in a split second and the appropriate response, such as telling us to remove our hand from a hot stove, protects and maintains that organ or tissue in good condition.

D. D. Palmer explained the spine's special role in aiding nerve impulses in *The Science, Art and Philosophy of Chiropractic (The Chiropractor's Adjuster).* Because it contains and protects the cord through which nerve impulses flow, the spinal column is vital. *Subluxations* of the vertebrae could impinge upon the branching nerves, reducing their ability to supply the organ or tissue with the correct amount of energy to function properly. He wrote:

> Displacement of any part of the skeletal frame may press against nerves, which are channels of communication, intensifying or decreasing their carrying capacity, creating either too much or not enough functioning, an aberration know as disease. The nature of the affection depends on the shape of the bone, the amount of pressure, age of patient, character of nerves impinged upon and individual make-up.

THE BODY WISDOM OF CHIROPRACTIC: INNATE INTELLIGENCE

Though Palmer's theory is now accepted by modern science, it was considered highly unorthodox in 1895. With it, he introduced an even more radical concept which continues to be a source of controversy: that of *innate intelligence.* Its theory and function form the cornerstone of chiropractic philosophy today.

Innate intelligence is variously known in Western thought as inborn wisdom, body wisdom, the God within, organism consciousness, and living force. Millions of people sense the presence of innate intelligence though it cannot be measured by scientific instruments. It is that part of us which directs the liver to perform more than 500 different functions in 24 hours without our conscious thought. It stands behind our instinct to survive and adapt to a changing environment, directing the body to heal itself when sick or injured. Our ability to make wise judgments according to the rules of common sense is also guided by innate intelligence. D. D. Palmer explained it in the following way: "There is an inborn intelligence in every living being, and in every plant that grows. Innate uses the sympathetic nervous system as channels through which to transmit its orders. . . . Innate has all to do with the control of the vital functions, and through them, indirectly, the control of the intellectual functions."

Its complement is *educated intelligence.* B. J. Palmer wrote: "The intelligence of the educated mind is wholly acquired—learned by experience. The innate is not acquired. It is born within us and with us, and is capable of running all functions of the body at birth as in adult life."

Chiropractic promotes a profound respect for the inborn wisdom which the body houses. For this reason, the goal is not to stimulate or inhibit the workings of the innate like those who use drugs, heat, cold, manipulation, or surgery, but rather to remove interference so that inborn wisdom can perform, unimpeded, the task of keeping the body healthy.

THE ROLE OF THE CHIROPRACTOR: THE DEBATE

D. D. Palmer defined the practitioner's unique, specialized role as locating, analyzing, and removing subluxations. "Chiropractors adjust, by hand, all displacements of the 200 bones, more especially those of the vertebral column, for the purposes of removing nerve impingements which are the cause of deranged functions."

B. J. Palmer affirmed his father's contention at first, but later refined its scope to include only the vertebrae of the spine. "Chiropractors limit practice to the adjustment, by hand only, of the articulations of the human spinal column for the purpose of removing interference to the transmission of nerve energy between brain and body." He underscored preventive chiropractic as "a philosophy, science and art of all things natural; a system of adjusting the segments of the spine by hand for the correction of the cause of dis-ease."

Like his father, B. J. was strict in his particular approach known as *straight chiropractic.* Limiting attention to the human spine was *the* feature making the new science separate and distinct from other health care systems. His most controversial stand defined the primary task of the chiropractor as involving neither diagnosis nor treatment of disease:

> Chiropractic is a science of the cause of things natural; not a science of symptoms; not a science of how to treat them; not a science to chemically analyze the constituents of the human body (normal or abnormal). But it is the science of how to analyze certain conditions quickly back to the cause, and we only utilize conditions in so far as they exist as a guidepost or mile-post on the road, telling us purely which way we must go.

Today, many practitioners (known as "straights") maintain this conservative position, devoting their preventive efforts to manual adjustments of the vertebral column, but the majority (dubbed "mixers" by D. D. Palmer) do not. They feel that the scope of chiropractic should include various methods of treatment like acupressure, soft tissue manipulation (massage), heat, and electrotherapy which assist in the healing process and in relieving pain. Therefore, several broader definitions of chiropractic have evolved.

Contemporary Chiropractic Philosophy

The following points are the core of the profession's current philosophical framework:

1. The nervous system is of paramount importance in the body's ability to maintain itself in good health.
2. Nerve interference is a primary factor in disease (dis-ease).
3. Spinal segments, or vertebrae, may become misaligned.
4. This misalignment will either directly or indirectly alter nerve messages to or from the brain, which can result in control center (brain) misinterpretation of proper function.
5. A force applied to the spine in the opposite direction of the misalignment will allow the body's inherent recuperative powers to realign the appropriate spinal segment. The repositioning of the vertebra will result in a reduction of nerve interference, which will directly or indirectly affect the functioning of the nervous system as a whole.
6. The primary goal of the chiropractor is to adjust spinal misalignments with the intention of removing nerve interference so that optimum nerve function can be restored.

CHIROPRACTIC: WHAT IT'S NOT

Many people confuse chiropractic with osteopathy, as well as with certain adjuncts to chiropractic like acupressure and massage. To help clarify the situation, let's review the definition and history of each.

Osteopathy

Chiropractic and osteopathy are often confused with each other, and with good reason:

> Each holds that structural derangements, especially of the spine, can lead to ill health.
>
> Both seek to realign those bones to their normal position in order to restore normal body functions.

Osteopathy was founded in 1874 by Andrew Taylor Still, a physician from Kansas City, Missouri. A. T. Still's basic premise was a simple one: the body cannot function properly unless it is structurally sound. He maintained that "all diseases are mere effects, the cause being a partial or complete failure of the nerves to properly conduct the fluids of life." He insisted that the secret to health lay in the liberation and purification of the bloodstream. As long as the blood was flowing normally, disease could not take hold. This "rule of the artery" is one feature that sets it apart from chiropractic, which concentrates on nerve interference.

Both the osteopath and chiropractor work with misaligned bones; it is in approach that they differ. While chiropractic stresses manual adjustments characterized by the dynamic thrust of specific vertebrae, osteopathic manipulation is a more generalized procedure which includes leverage, traction, and pressure in order to correct abnormal structure. In addition, osteopaths employ other techniques to eliminate symptoms and mobilize the body's inherent resistance to disease. These include massage, stretching, twisting, and the application of water (hydrotherapy) or heat.

Both D. D. and B. J. Palmer were upset by the confusion of the two. In his colorful style, B. J. expressed the major differences in his textbook *The Science of Chiropractic:*

> The osteopath, by rubbing, kneading, pressing, and a general overhauling, by neck-twisting, arm and leg

> wrings, aims to inhibit or stimulate nerves, whip up circulation, slow up or stimulate the action of the heart and other organs. The M.D.'s try to produce precisely the same effect by drugs. Chiropractors never deaden, inhibit or stimulate nerves, or the vital organs of the body; they free nerves from impingement, so that their impulses may be normal.

Still's claims of 100 percent cures and his inability to explain to the satisfaction of those in traditional medicine how osteopathy worked resulted in its banishment—like chiropractic—into professional exile, far adrift from the mainstream of medical practice.

After Dr. Still's death, refinements and modifications of his original ideas were introduced. Osteopathy slowly began moving closer to orthodox medicine by placing more emphasis on drugs and less on spinal manipulations until it is now a respected part of the medical mainstream. Modern therapy can include surgery, physiotherapy, radium treatment, diets, and vitamins and drugs.

Acupressure (*Shiatsu*)

Acupressure (known as *Shiatsu* in Japan) is closely related to acupuncture but involves applying firm pressure of the fingertips to specific contact points (of which there are 102) rather than puncturing them with needles.

Often used along with chiropractic, it is not necessarily compatible with the former's basic approach to health. Both systems work with the inherent recuperative forces of the body, but acupressure—like acupuncture—works to stimulate the flow of energy to organs and tissues. The chiropractor's main goal is not to inhibit or stimulate but to remove nerve interference on a fundamental level so innate intelligence can send nerve impulses unimpeded to all the body's organs and tissues.

Touch for Health

One recent development in the health field is Touch for Health, a form of preventive care developed in 1970 by a chiropractor from California, Dr. John F. Thie.

Touch for Health does not diagnose or treat specific diseases. It helps locate and correct imbalances in the body's energy system through applied kinesiology to related muscles of the body's twelve major organs. For example, the tester puts pressure on an arm or leg while the subject resists. If the subject cannot resist, the related organ is determined to be weak. Firm pressure is then applied to the appropriate reflex point, stimulating the weakened area. After several moments, the muscle is retested.

Touch for Health is sometimes confused with chiropractic because applied kinesiology is sometimes used to evaluate the effectiveness of adjustments. After the first muscle test, an adjustment is given. A follow up test can determine if it has helped the organ regain a normal level of function.

Massage

People have a popular misconception that chiropractic is a form of massage. Though sometimes used as an adjunct to chiropractic adjustments, the two are different.

The person skilled in massage works with soft tissues like muscles, fatty tissue, and skin. A masseur or masseuse is trained in the art of kneading, slapping, rolling, pressing, and stroking these soft tissues to enable the body's self-healing process to take place. It is possible that massage can remove nerve interference although that is not its major goal.

Some chiropractors use it in addition to adjustments while others hire certified massage therapists to treat their patients.

ALLOPATHY AND CHIROPRACTIC: COMPARING THE BASICS

The principle of allopathy is one of the simplest known to humanity. It makes up the foundation of the medical profession today. Unlike chiropractic and other health systems, allopathy maintains that when the body's workings deviate from normal, a counteracting procedure should be applied. For example, an allopath would give you an alkaline for acid indigestion, a sleeping pill to treat insomnia, or a cold compress to reduce a fever.

Chiropractic seeks to remove any underlying nerve interference which can hamper the body's natural healing process. While allopathic medicine holds that germs and harmful bacteria are the primary cause of disease, chiropractic maintains that a body which is unhealthy in the first place is vulnerable to bacteria and germs. The former prescribes a wide variety of drugs to inhibit or stimulate normal body functions. The latter does not. These important differences are reflected both in the nature and quality of health care we pay for in each case.

Doctors of Cause Versus Doctors of Therapy

An enthusiastic woman told me her chiropractor had cured her arthritis. When I talked to him later, he would not take credit for healing her painful, swollen joints. I asked him to explain why and received the simple answer, "Because we chiropractors don't cure disease." He said professional healers never cure disease. Only the body possesses the ability to heal itself. His task is to merely help the body do its job by removing any interference to the natural healing process.

Most medical doctors would agree, citing that some 80

percent of all disease is self-limiting. That means the body will cure the problem without any treatment at all. The chiropractor made a further point: Although he relieves pain and other disease symptoms in the course of his practice, he is primarily a doctor of *cause* while others are doctors of *therapy*. A chiropractor uses symptoms as a guidepost to a deeper problem (i.e. the cause). The medical doctor devotes most of his attention to treating the symptoms themselves.

Headache, for example, is a symptom. Traditional doctors use the therapy-oriented approach, prescribing pain killing drugs to relieve the ache. This may help us feel better, but the drug is covering the pain while the basic cause remains undetected. In this case, pain is a valuable indication telling us something is wrong (lack of sleep, nervous tension, or a vertebral subluxation) yet this important inner voice is silenced.

Constipation is another common symptom treated by therapy. When it occurs, we take a laxative to force the body to eliminate waste. Most laxatives work by irritating the bowel and the body rejects them along with fecal matter. Unfortunately, the intestinal flora—so vitally needed for proper digestion—are often lost with the laxative and waste.

How would chiropractors treat a headache or constipation? They wouldn't specifically. Because chiropractic is primarily intended to treat not symptoms but causes, adjustments would remove interference, enabling the body to resume proper flow of nerve energy to the affected organ. Normal functioning results. In addition, such factors as diet, exercise, and stress may be analyzed to see how they may contribute to these disorders and what can be done to modify their effect.

How We "Get Sick"

Since the mid-nineteenth century, the medical profession has maintained that most illness is caused by germs, harmful bacteria, and virus transmitted to people through food, breath, and touch. Our language reflects this idea as in "catching" a cold, "coming down with a bug," or "it's been going around."

Although it may be true that many of us are susceptible to various strains of bacteria and virus, chiropractic maintains that germs do not open the door to disease. *Dis-ease and ill health open the door to germs.* B. J. Palmer pointed out that if germs were as dangerous as we thought, nobody would be left to worry about them, since we are constantly breathing, eating, drinking, and touching germs everywhere, 24 hours a day.

No responsible practitioner would guarantee that chiropractic care would give immunity to all germs and disease. It is an established fact, however, that healthy people are far less susceptible to disease than unhealthy people.

Instead of blaming illness on germs, or "bad luck," chiropractic helps the patient take control by insuring a strong nerve supply to every part of the body. This energy flow helps maintain all tissue cells in good health. It regulates the body's production of natural antibodies which destroy harmful bacteria. As health is maintained without vaccines or other drugs, a germ or virus does not have fertile ground in which to sustain itself.

A Pill for Every Ill . . .

According to a recent issue of the *Social Security Bulletin*, Americans spend over $4 billion a year on 7000 different nonprescription drugs. In addition to these over-the-counter pharmaceutical purchases, the public spends over $11 billion on prescription drugs, or 7.7 prescriptions filled per person each year.

Chiropractors do not prescribe drugs, but they believe certain medications are necessary to save a life or maintain certain body functions when all else fails. The chiropractic profession is strongly opposed to those medical doctors and drug companies, however, who proclaim they've got "a pill for every ill and a potion for every emotion" and that it is perfectly all right to take a drug for every little thing that comes along.

In the United States and other industrialized nations, central nervous system drugs (barbiturates, tranquilizers, and amphetamines) represent the fastest growing sector of the pharmaceutical industry, amounting to one-third of the total sales. Chiropractors are concerned about the possible effects stimulants and tranquilizers have on the nervous system's ability to maintain the body in optimum physical and mental condition. In addition, they question the overall negative side effects which drugs may have on the body.

Another concern involves dangerous *synergistic* effects which occur when two or more drugs combine in the body to produce a chemical reaction. An example of this made headlines in 1977 after the sudden death of Elvis Presley. According to a medical examiner's report, ten prescription drugs were present in the singer's bloodstream when he died. The synergistic reaction they produced contributed to his death.

For the majority of individuals, drugs are habitually taken in order to relieve unpleasant symptoms. Chiropractic teaches that they only suppress or alter symptoms and body functions. A fever is one way the body fights off infection. If an aspirin is taken to reduce it, our body's ability to combat the infection is reduced.

Chiropractors believe that lack of sleep, emotional stress, improper diet, smoking, lack of exercise, overeating, alcohol consumption, and especially subluxations of the spine are the major causes of pain and other symptoms. For this reason, chiropractors work with nature to help normalize proper body function. Drugs cover up symptoms, cause physical and psychological dependency, or have possible side effects. Chiropractic teaches that a move away from drugs toward the natural ability of the body to heal itself will have a positive, lasting effect on our health which will be passed on to future generations.

4

Chiropractic: Working with Your Nervous System and Spine

DANIEL DAVID PALMER WAS RIDICULED BY MEMbers of the medical profession when he said the normally functioning brain, operating through a sound nervous system, regulates and integrates every body activity down to the workings of the tiniest cell. Today, his theory on which chiropractic is based is universally accepted by the scientific community and is taught in every medical school in the country.

Each organ of the body receives its vital nerve supply from the brain via the spinal cord and nerve trunks. If the supply is interfered with, an increase or decrease of nerve energy to the organ or tissue can result. Because the central nervous system is housed by the spinal column, communicating with every part of the body from it, the science of chiropractic has specifically concerned itself with spinal structure. It investigates how misalignments alter functions of the central nervous system, leading to ill health. Understanding how to correct nerve interference and restore proper energy transmission to the entire body is the chief goal of chiropractic research. A lay person's knowledge of the nervous system can help you become a partner with your chiropractor in maintaining your health.

The *autonomic nervous system* is responsible for carrying out the involuntary processes of the body such as digestion, repair, and elimination. Without our conscious thought it adjusts the functions of the muscles and the internal organs to the advantage of the organism as a whole.

Within the autonomic nervous system, two sets of nerves generally work opposite each other to regulate *homeostasis* or body balance. For example, one set (known as the sympathetic nervous system) speeds up the heart and slows down digestion, while the other set (the parasympathetic nervous system) slows down the heart and speeds up digestion. Together, with utmost precision, they regulate the body's functions and keep them in perfect balance.

The *central nervous system* is composed of the brain, spinal cord, and nerves as they exit from the spine. It is responsible for helping the body adapt to its external environment as in locomotion and the ability to sense our surroundings.

Both systems are interconnected by way of the spinal nerves. Any predisposing condition or obstruction in one system can alter the normal function of the other. A simplified drawing reveals the major divisions. Their relationship to important body organs can be seen in Figure 4–1.

BRAIN, SPINE, AND NERVES: A TEAM EFFORT

The central nervous system is of special interest to the practitioner who works to keep it free of interference. It begins in the brain, which contains countless billions of *neurons* or nerve

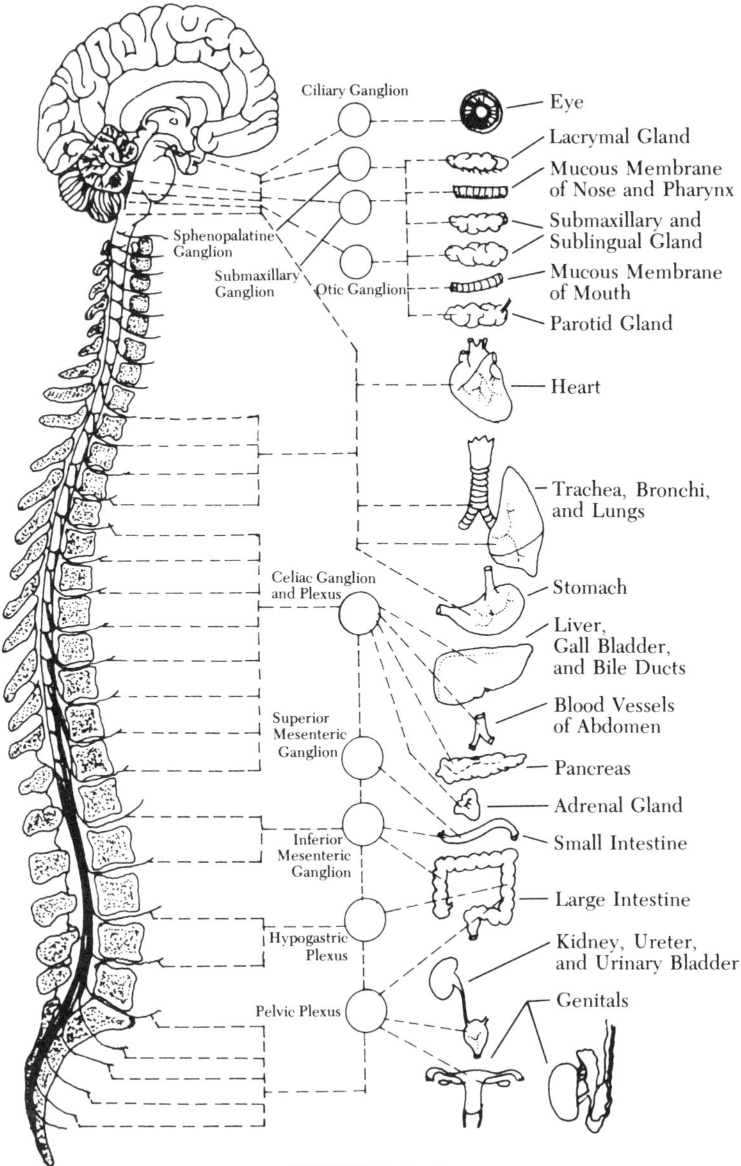

FIGURE 4–1

The nervous system, revealing two divisions: central and autonomic. From Schafer, *Chiropractic Health Care*. Reprinted courtesy of The Foundation for Chiropractic Education and Research.

cells that transmit information from one part of the nervous system to another.

From the base of the brain, the spinal cord extends through the spinal column (Figure 4–1). The brain uses it as a pathway through which it controls and governs the function of every organ and tissue of the body. Just as the brain is protected by a reinforced shield of bone (the skull), nature has given the spinal cord special protection as well. Its first line of defense is the spinal column composed of a long series of bones called vertebrae. These encase the spinal cord and protect it from injury. *Cerebrospinal fluid* flows within the coverings of the cord. Although we don't know everything about this unique fluid, we do know it is vital to the transmission of nerve impulses and proper nourishment and cleansing of delicate nerve tissue.

Thirty-one pairs of nerves branch out from the spinal column. Each is made of billions of fibers less than 1/100th the size of a human hair. Each nerve trunk passes through an opening called the *intervertebral foramen,* which is located between the vertebrae (Figure 4–2). This is the critical juncture where a misalignment can impinge on a nerve trunk and affect normal nerve transmission. In addition to the spinal nerves, our bodies contain twelve pairs of cranial nerves, which include the optic, acoustic, facial, and nasal nerves, which radiate to the eyes, ears, face, and nose (including the jaw), and the vagus nerve, which passes through the neck and chest to the upper part of the abdomen.

Although cranial nerves work independently from spinal nerves, chiropractic takes note of them for they, too, are affected by alterations in the blood supply. They receive transmissions from bundles of relay stations (known as ganglia) which are directly connected to the spinal nerves. For this reason, health problems relating to ear, eye, and nasal passages are known to respond favorably to chiropractic adjustments.

Through this marvelous network of nerves, the brain re-

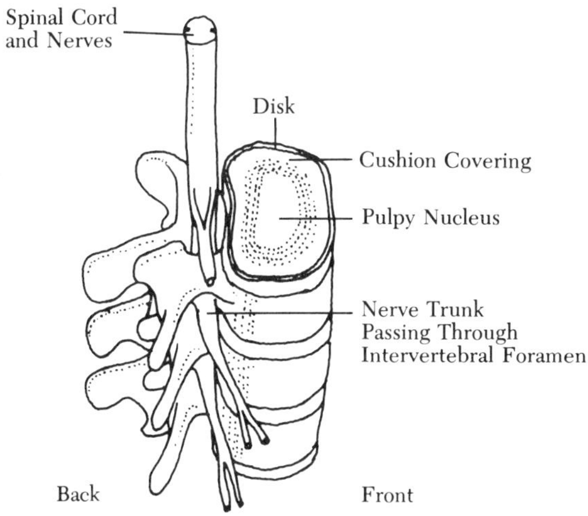

FIGURE 4–2

Detailed section of the lumbar spine, showing the relationship between spinal nerves and spinal column.

sponds to and controls the function of every cell in the body. When the nervous system is free of interference, good health is the result. But when interference due to misalignment exists, a state of dis-ease may occur.

DISRUPTION OF THE NERVOUS SYSTEM: A CASE HISTORY

The relationship between the spine and the nervous system is extremely complex. Chiropractic research has determined that even the slightest misalignment can produce nerve interference which may surface with a variety of effects. According to Dr. Frank P. DeGiacomo of the New York Chiropractic College, "Anatomical disrelation either macroscopic or microscopic may disturb the normal generation, transmission, distribution or expression of the nervous system, and may cause symptoms or pathology local to or remote from the particular region." This means that nerve interference may produce immediate or cumulative effects on any part of the body.

For example, an impinged nerve in the lower thoracic (midback) area may cause localized pain or weakness in an organ the nerve services, such as the colon. Constipation, spasticity, or colitis may result immediately or after a period of time. Impairment of the proper flow of energy through a nerve is usually followed by a malfunction in the organ which it services.

Let's examine the case histories of two college athletes, Charles S. and Roy B. Both were slightly injured during the football season one year and received similar subluxations in the thoracic area of their spines. For Charles, the nerve impingement produced back pain, making it difficult to play on the team or even attend classes. After several days of extreme discomfort, he sought out a local chiropractor who adjusted his spine, removing the cause of nerve interference. Within five minutes the pain was gone. The following Monday, Charles was back on the team.

Roy, on the other hand, felt nothing and continued to play on the football team. Eighteen months later, however, he began to suffer from intestinal problems. (The intestine is one of the organs fed by the impinged thoracic nerve.) Although the university health service gave medication to relieve chronic constipation and intestinal cramps, Roy's health did not improve. His teammate, Charles, suggested he visit his chiropractor. Roy soon received a series of chiropractic adjustments for several weeks (three per week for three weeks). The nerve supply to his intestinal organs was normalized and symptoms soon began to diminish.

According to the Commission of Inquiry in New Zealand, chiropractors are the only health practitioners equipped by education and training to carry out the specialized task of removing nerve interference with chiropractic spinal adjustments.

THE SPINE: YOUR PILLAR OF LIFE

Long before Hippocrates, a healthy spine was recognized as vital to good health. Today, chiropractic is the only science specifically concerned with proper care of the spine and the relationship between it and the nervous system.

The spinal column, the main shaft of the body, is composed of twenty-four movable bones called vertebrae (from the Latin word *vertere:* to turn). The spine joins at the base with the sacrum and coccyx. By the time we reach adulthood, the sacrum and coccyx fuse into bones with no movement between their segments. There are four principle groups of vertebrae (Figure 4–3). The seven most superior are the *cervical* vertebrae which make up the neck. They are followed by twelve more in the upper and midback known as the *thoracic* (or dorsal) vertebrae. The five below them are called *lumbar* vertebrae, the largest and heaviest bones of the spinal column. They support the weight of the entire upper half of the body. Of special interest to chiropractors, misalignments of the lumbar vertebrae are often responsible for painful disc problems and other low back conditions. Inferior to the lumbar are *sacral* vertebrae, which in turn are followed by the coccyx made of four or five tiny bones. The latter appear to be a remnant of a tail, and for that reason are often referred to as the tailbone.

Segments of the spine are arranged one upon the other forming a strong pillar. Hundreds of muscles attach to each one permitting free movement of the entire body.

Since we walk upright, the spinal column carries the weight of the entire trunk and head, withstanding constant jarring and stress.

To help maintain the integrity of the spinal column, nature has provided small cartilaginous cushions between the vertebrae known as *intervertebral discs.* These "shock absorbers" are carefully fitted so that jarring and strain have minimal effect on the spine and nervous system. However, these spinal discs are constantly subject to gravity and torque from body move-

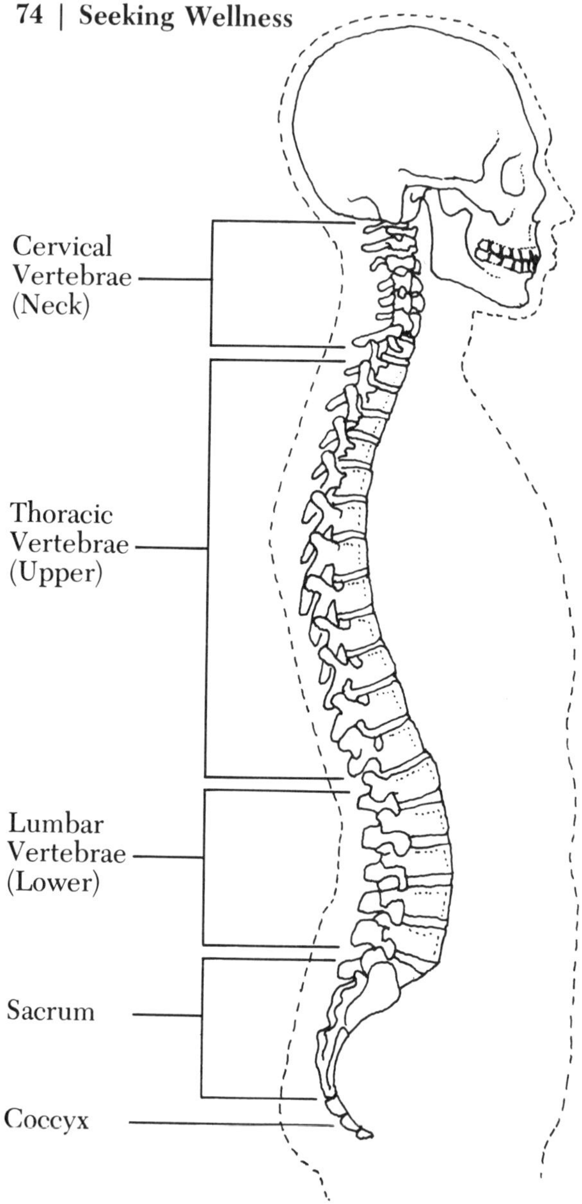

FIGURE 4–3

The spinal column. From Inglis, *The Book of the Back*. Reprinted courtesy of Ebury Press.

ments and are therefore susceptible to wear and tear over the years. Spinal misalignments caused by falls, automobile accidents, improper lifting, or sprains may allow the disc to "slip," bulge, herniate, or impinge upon delicate spinal nerves.

THE SUBLUXATION: AN OUT-OF-LINE RESPONSE

The spine is so beautifully designed that intervertebral foramina between the bones are exactly the correct shape and size to accommodate the big nerve trunks (along with veins and arteries) which pass through them. If openings are properly maintained, nerve energy from the brain flows freely through the nerve trunks and onward to eventually reach every cell of the body. But if one or more vertebrae are out of alignment, the opening becomes smaller as the result of a hard bone impinging on a soft nerve (Figure 4–4). According to the Federation of Straight Chiropractic Organization (FSCO) Constitution, a misaligned vertebrae, or *subluxation*, is defined as "A condition which a vertebra has lost its juxtaposition with the one above, the one below, or both, to the extent less than a luxation (dislocation); occluding an opening; impinging a nerve; and interfering with normal transmission of mental impulses between the brain and the tissue cells of the body."

Medical doctors often overlook the subtlety of subluxations, claiming that they are figments of the chiropractor's imagination. The fact they exist and have a powerful impact on health, however, has been documented in medical journals since 1909 (see Chapter 1). The distinguished surgeon James P. Warbasse, M.D., wrote: "Subluxations of the vertebrae occur in all parts of the spine and in all degrees. When the dislocation is so slight as not to affect the spinal cord, it will still produce disturbances in the spinal nerves, passing off through the spinal foramina."

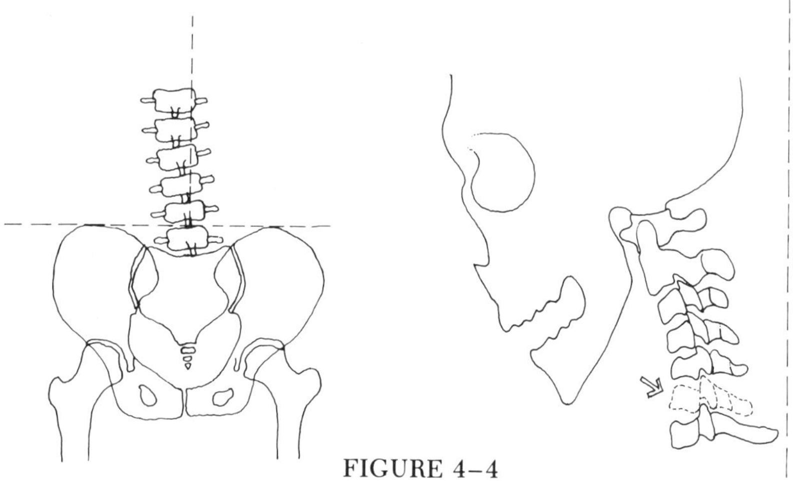

FIGURE 4–4

(Left) An abnormal curvature with several subluxations of the lower back. *(Right)* A subluxation of the sixth cervical vertebra. Note uneven disc space between vertebrae. From Schafer, *Chiropractic Health Care.* Reprinted courtesy of The Foundation for Chiropractic Education and Research.

A subluxation may be large enough to be recognized by the untrained eye or so small that it escapes the attention of everybody but the most experienced specialists. Recent studies have found that the degree of displacement has no direct correlation with the amount of nerve interference present. A tiny misalignment can inhibit the vital flow of the cerebrospinal fluid for impulse transmission. Therefore, most chiropractors will pay attention to a tiny subluxation which the medical doctor or physiotherapist would consider insignificant.

Regardless of the size of the subluxation, the resultant pressure and possible irritation of the delicate spinal nerves may *increase* or *decrease* the flow of nerve energy to the organs or tissues served by the nerve, causing a state of dis-ease. How energy flow is affected depends on the particular individual's reaction. It cannot be determined in advance. Most people have subluxations that go uncorrected for years. Although not immediately evident, an uncorrected misalignment can produce long term effects which may result in permanent damage to organs or to the spine itself, limiting movement and causing degeneration of vertebrae. When left uncorrected, a simple spinal misalignment can develop into a serious condition that can even result in death because nerve transmission is completely blocked off.

The Case of Henry M.

The following case history illustrates how an uncorrected subluxation can lead to a serious and complex state of dis-ease (Figure 4–5).

Henry M. suffered a major displacement in the midback when he took a bad fall on the ice while walking home from work. Although he felt severe pain for three weeks, he forgot about the incident as soon as the discomfort faded. The subluxation involved the fifth thoracic spinal nerve leading to the liver and solar plexus.

Henry appeared to enjoy reasonably good health for years, but his liver had begun to malfunction in regulating the amount of cholesterol in the blood. Henry's love for hamburgers and sausage didn't help. It forced the liver to work that much harder purifying the blood of toxic bacteria, antibiotics, and hormones found in the meat. Henry felt heavy and bloated even after a small meal and sometimes had to lie down while the liver slowly cleansed the blood.

Since the weakened organ was unable to function at peak efficiency, its ability to supply the brain with adequate amounts of oxygen and glucose (a sugar) was impaired. As a result, Henry often became irritable and had trouble sleeping. The liver's ability to store vitamins was also diminished, and the result was several vitamin deficiencies. By the time Henry was 50 years old, his cholesterol count and blood pressure had reached dangerous levels and he was a frequent visitor to the local hospital for tests and medical treatment.

By the time Henry finally consulted a chiropractor, he

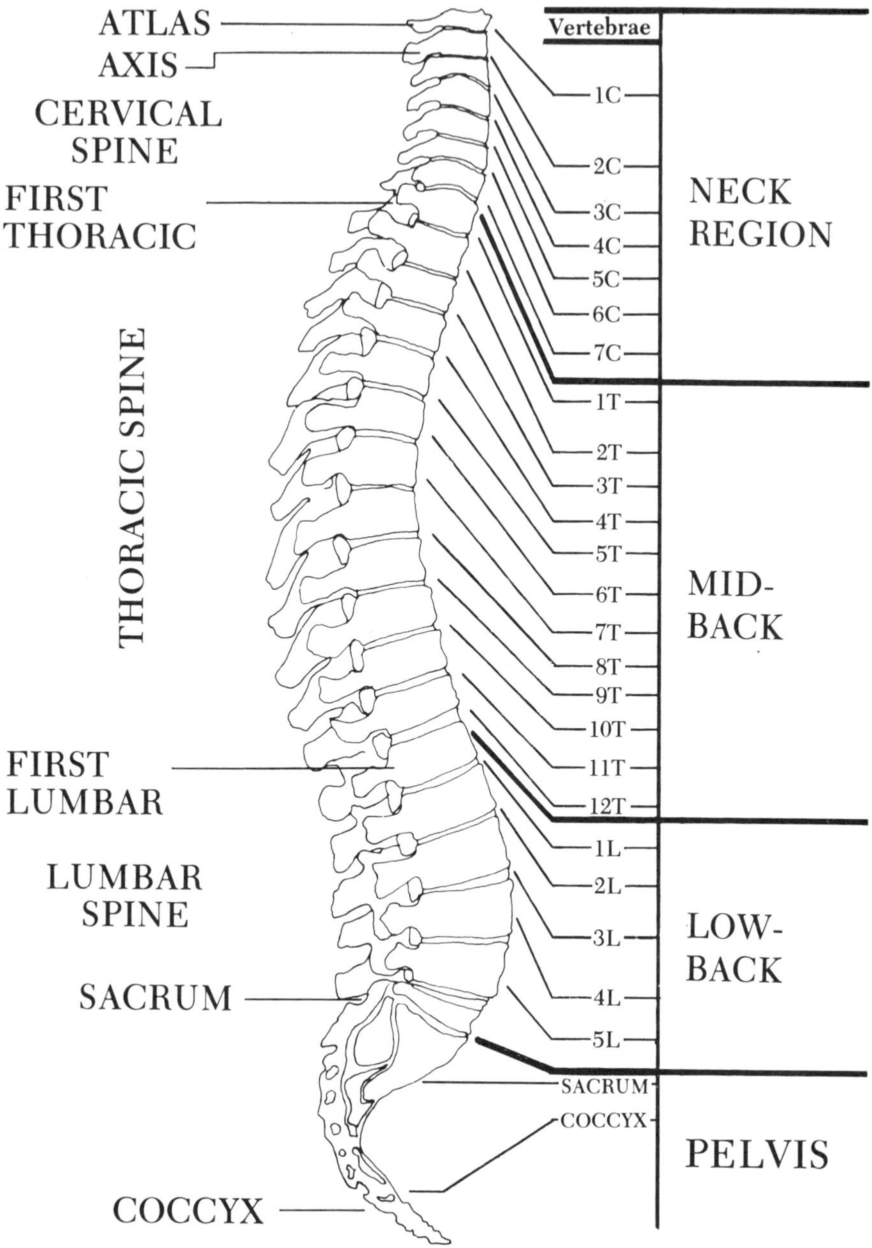

FIGURE 4–5

Chart of effects of spinal misalignments. "The nervous system controls and coordinates all organs and structures of the human body" (*Gray's Anatomy*, 29th ed., p. 4). Misalignments of spinal vertebrae

Areas	Effects
1C Blood supply to the head, pituitary gland, scalp, bones of the face, brain, inner and middle ear, sympathetic nervous system.	Headaches, nervousness, insomnia, head colds, high blood pressure, migraine headaches, nervous breakdowns, amnesia, chronic tiredness, dizziness.
2C Eyes, optic nerves, auditory nerves, sinuses, mastoid bones, tongue, forehead.	Sinus trouble, allergies, crossed eyes, deafness, eye troubles, earache, fainting spells, certain cases of blindness.
3C Cheeks, outer ear, face bones, teeth, trifacial nerve.	Neuralgia, neuritis, acne or pimples, eczema.
4C Nose, lips, mouth, eustachian tube.	Hay fever, catarrh, hearing loss, adenoids.
5C Vocal cords, neck glands, pharnyx.	Laryngitis, hoarseness, throat conditions such as sore throat or quinsy.
6C Neck muscles, shoulders, tonsils.	Stiff neck, pain in upper arm, tonsilitis, whooping cough, croup.
7C Thyroid gland, bursae in the shoulders, elbows.	Bursitis, colds, thyroid conditions.
1T Arms from elbows down, including hands, wrists, fingers; esophagus and trachea.	Asthma, cough, difficult breathing, shortness of breath, pain in lower arms and hands.
2T Heart, including its valves and covering; coronary arteries.	Functional heart conditions and certain chest conditions.
3T Lungs, bronchial tubes, chest, breast.	Bronchitis, pleurisy, pneumonia, congestion, influenza.
4T Gall bladder, common duct.	Gall bladder conditions, jaundice, shingles.
5T Liver, solar plexus, blood.	Liver conditions, fevers, low blood pressure, anemia, poor circulation, arthritis.
6T Stomach.	Stomach troubles, including nervous stomach; indigestion, heartburn, dyspepsia.
7T Pancreas, duodenum.	Ulcers, gastritis.
8T Spleen, diaphragm.	Hiccoughs, lowered resistance.
9T Adrenal and supra-renal glands.	Allergies, hives.
10T Kidneys	Kidney troubles, hardening of the arteries, chronic tiredness, nephritis, pyelitis.
11T Kidneys, ureters.	Skin conditions such as acne, pimples, eczema, or boils.
12T Small intestines, lymph circulation.	Rheumatism, gas pains, certain types of sterility.
1L Large intestines, inguinal rings.	Constipation, colitis, dysentery, diarrhea, some ruptures or hernias.
2L Appendix, abdomen, upper leg.	Cramps, difficult breathing, acidosis, varicose veins.
3L Sex organs, uterus, bladder, knees.	Bladder troubles, menstrual troubles such as painful or irregular periods, miscarriages, bed wetting, impotency, change of life symptoms, many knee pains.
4L Prostate gland, muscles of the lower back, sciatic nerve.	Sciatica; lumbago; difficult, painful, or too frequent urination; backaches.
5L Lower legs, ankles, feet.	Poor circulation in the legs, swollen ankles, weak ankles and arches, cold feet, weakness in the legs, leg cramps.
SACRUM Hip bones, buttocks.	Sacro-iliac conditions, spinal curvatures.
COCCYX Rectum, anus.	Hemorrhoids (piles), pruritis (itching), pain at end of spine on sitting.

and discs may cause irritation to the nervous system and affect the structures, organs, and functions, which may result in the conditions shown above. Reprinted courtesy of the Parker Chiropractic Research Foundation.

looked and felt twenty years older than his age, and was a prime candidate for a stroke or heart attack. The chiropractor located the misalignment that was contributing to his trouble and adjusted it. Fortunately for Henry, the subluxation could still be healed by the body. After six weeks of care, he began to feel much better, although not all body functions had returned to normal. The damage was done, but long-term chances for reclaiming health were good.

Most people aren't as fortunate as Henry M. They ignore the potential effects of a vertebral subluxation, opening the door to a state of dis-ease which may lead to chronic degenerative illness, or even death.

THE SUBLUXATION: REDUCING RISK

Subluxations are very common phenomena. We receive dozens of them every day. Although some cause pain, most do not and are beyond our awareness. The vast majority are corrected through normal spinal movement when we stretch and move about during the day. There are three basic ways the spine can become misaligned, which can be traced to chemical, psychological, and mechanical causes. By becoming aware of these causes, we can reduce the risk of subluxation, consulting a chiropractor for a spinal examination when we experience one of them.

Beware: Our Chemical Environment

After suffering an allergic reaction to an antibiotic, Diane S. felt mild back pain. Her chiropractor believed the subluxation he discovered after a spinal examination may have been due to the adverse drug reaction.

David C. just returned from a visit to Mexico, where the drinking water in a particular village made him ill. Although he wasn't aware of it, his body's reaction to the water brought about a vertebral misalignment.

John K. visits a chiropractor every week, and his doctor always notices that he has an abnormally high amount of subluxations to correct. He is certain that John's chronic cigarette smoking is a major cause.

Daniel David Palmer was probably the first person to call attention to the importance of chemical irritants and toxins as major causes of spinal misalignments. Discussing them in his textbook, he wrote: "The poison, acting on certain nerves, irritates their structure. They in turn contract muscles which draw vertebrae out of alignment, thereby impinging upon nerves which go and affect certain portions of the body."

Fifty years later, a book written exclusively about spinal misalignments (*The Neurodynamics of the Vertebral Subluxation* by Dr. A. E. Homewood) cited dozens of medical studies which substantiate Palmer's claim that solid, liquid, or gaseous toxins from food additives, tobacco, exhaust fumes, other environmental pollution, or drugs may cause nerves to react so that body structures, such as the muscles, can be affected enough to move a vertebra out of alignment.

Although chiropractic cannot claim to eliminate the risk of environmental contamination, periodic adjustments help our bodies resist the modern chemical environment.

Beware: Our Emotional Environment

Greg T. rushed to catch the 8 o'clock flight to Chicago. He gave himself plenty of time, but an accident on the freeway caused a mammoth traffic jam. After hectic driving on detours and side streets, he reached the boarding gate with only minutes to spare. As he collapsed exhaustedly into his seat,

Greg realized his head was pounding and his neck was stiff. The headache was gone by the time the plane touched down in Chicago, but the subluxation he suffered was not. After a month of low-grade neck pain, Greg consulted a chiropractor who removed the pressure on a cervical nerve with a single painless adjustment.

If you have indigestion or suffer from an ingrown toenail, the pain affects your mental state and may put you in a bad mood. By the same token, a state of mind can make you ill, as Greg T.'s case illustrates. Medical science has documented that fear, rage, depression, and emotional shock can produce a variety of pathological conditions like sudden death or *psychosomatic disease,* which is illness caused by mental or emotional stress.

Chiropractors maintain that feelings can bring about spinal subluxations. In his work to integrate the human body with psychiatry, Wilhelm Reich found that people retract their pelvic area in response to shame, fear, or anxiety about sex. The abnormal posture created over a long period of time produces compensatory changes in body structure which accents the primary and secondary curves of the spine. Dr. A. E. Homewood, former president of the Canadian Memorial Chiropractic College in Toronto, wrote that chronic muscular tension may contribute to localized subluxations which could become major if left uncorrected.

As stated in Chapter 1, chiropractic is not a panacea for emotional disorders, but it can help us achieve a state of good mental health. By freeing our bodies of nerve interference, a major cause of internal stress is removed. As a result, a person is not only relieved of tension, but can adapt more easily to stress and function at a higher level of efficiency and emotional balance. By breaking the vicious circle of subluxation, pain, and emotional pressure, the chiropractor helps us enjoy a benign circle of vitality, adaptability, and emotional wellbeing.

Beware: Our Physical Environment

Peter M. stood in line waiting for tickets to a concert when he sneezed. Immediately he felt something "go" in his back and could barely walk. After three chiropractic adjustments, Peter was able to walk again without a twinge of pain.

Linda B. broke two ribs in a serious car accident. She also felt a tingling in her left leg which the medical doctor felt was linked to spinal nerve trauma. After four months of chiropractic care, proper nerve transmission was restored to her leg and the tingling stopped.

George K. pulled some back muscles when he lifted a large box of tiles at work. The pain subsided after two days of heat treatments, but the subluxation wasn't detected until he saw a chiropractor for a routine visit three weeks later.

Millions of people suffer from subluxations related to chemical and emotional causes, but the case histories of misalignments due to physical trauma reflect the majority of patients who consult a chiropractor. Accidents, serious or minor, are the most common cause of mechanical subluxation. Slipping on the ice, falling off a bicycle or motorbike, or suffering a whiplash injury in a car accident may result in a spinal misalignment impinging on a nerve. Shovelling snow, moving heavy furniture, and improper lifting (such as bending over and stretching to remove a sack of groceries from the trunk or back seat of a car) are also major causes of subluxation.

Many ordinary tasks performed during a normal working day place repeated and prolonged strain on the spine and connecting muscles. Dentists, for example, are constantly stooping to perform dental work on their patients. Taxi drivers and truckers spend most of their time sitting in unnatural positions in seats of poor orthopedic design which lack proper back support. Mail carriers often make their rounds with a large sack weighing heavily on one shoulder. Auto mechanics and plumbers work in cramped, uncomfortable spaces. Farmers, carpenters, secretaries, miners, athletes, dancers, and even writers work at jobs which produce stress and strain on the spine.

Of all occupations, however, homemaking is subjected to the widest variety of hazards such as lifting and carrying heavy packages and children, moving furniture, and turning mattresses. Practically every job produces some unnatural strain on the spinal column which can result in misalignment.

When we hear a small "click" or "pop" when we stretch, a minor displacement is being corrected. But those of a more serious nature (caused by accidents, strains, strong emotional reactions, or toxins) are not easily corrected by the body and, therefore, call for the attention of a professional.

There is general apprehension among prospective chiropractic patients, however. They do not know what a chiropractor is or how he or she is educated and licensed. The following chapter will explain what "makes a chiropractor" and explore how the practitioner becomes uniquely qualified to perform the exacting process of adjustments and be responsible for complete chiropractic care.

5

The Education of a Chiropractor

MODERN CHIROPRACTIC COLLEGES PROVIDE A high standard of specialized instruction not duplicated anywhere else. The regulations for chiropractic licensure in the United States and Canada define the limits to the chiropractor's domain. Throughout the world professional organizations are working to maintain the highest level of competence within chiropractic. Let's see what this means to us as health care consumers.

THE BACKBONE OF CHIROPRACTIC: EDUCATION

Over the last thirty years, education in the profession has experienced a major transformation. The nineteen training colleges in the United States, Canada, England, and Australia offer courses, facilities, and instructors of the highest calibre. The Congress of Education was established in 1947 by what is now the American Chiropractic Association. When the results of a study showed that the majority of practitioners wanted to improve the standard of chiropractic education to a uniform level that would qualify their accrediting agency for Department of Health, Education and Welfare approval, an ambitious campaign to achieve high educational standards was begun by the chiropractic profession itself.

As a result, a number of colleges had to close their doors and merge with stronger chiropractic institutions. Today, many schools are the result of two or three mergers. No large foundations, no drug companies, no government agencies gave money toward chiropractic education, yet college standards improved dramatically. On August 24, 1974, the Council of Chiropractic Education (CCE) was recognized by the U.S. Office of Education of the Department of Health, Education and Welfare as a valid accrediting agency for chiropractic colleges.

At the time of this writing, all but two schools enjoy membership status with the CCE. The others have chosen to establish an accrediting agency they feel is more qualified to set standards for a more conservative education. The following is a 1981 listing of all the chiropractic educational institutions in the United States, Canada, England, and Australia:

UNITED STATES

Adio Institute of Straight Chiropractic*
P.O. Box 849, Levittown, Pennsylvania 19058

Cleveland Chiropractic College
6401 Rockhill Road, Kansas City, Missouri 64131

Cleveland Chiropractic College
590 N. Vermont Avenue, Los Angeles, California 90004

* Not affiliated with CCE.

Life Chiropractic College
1269 Barclay Circle, Marietta, Georgia 30062

Logan College of Chiropractic
1851 Schoettler Road, Chesterfield, Missouri 63017

Los Angeles College of Chiropractic
920 E. Broadway, Glendale, California 91205

National Chiropractic College
200 E. Roosevelt Road, Lombard, Illinois 60148

New York Chiropractic College
P.O. Box 167, Glen Head, New York 11545

Northern California College of Chiropractic
1095 Dunford Way, Sunnyvale, California 94087

Northwestern College of Chiropractic
1834 S. Mississippi River Road, St. Paul, Minnesota 55116

Pacific States Chiropractic College
879 Grant Avenue, San Lorenzo, California 94580

Palmer College of Chiropractic
1000 Brady Street, Davenport, Iowa 52803

Pasadena College of Chiropractic
55 N. St. John Avenue, Pasadena, California 91103

Sherman College of Straight Chiropractic*
P.O. Box 1452, Springfield Road, Spartanburg, South Carolina 29304

Texas Chiropractic College
5912 Spencer Highway, Pasadena, Texas 77505

Western States Chiropractic College
2900 N.E. 132nd Avenue, Portland, Oregon 97230

* Not affiliated with CCE.

CANADA

Canadian Memorial Chiropractic College
1900 Bayview Avenue, Toronto, Ontario M4G 3E6

ENGLAND

Anglo European College of Chiropractic
Cavendish Road, Bournemouth, Hampshire
BH1 1RA

AUSTRALIA

International College of Chiropractic
P.O. Box 96, Bundoora (Melbourne) Victoria 3083

CHIROPRACTIC EDUCATION TODAY: CURRICULUM QUALIFICATIONS

In most states, students of chiropractic are required to have earned sixty college credits (approximately two years) with special emphasis on biology, physics, and chemistry before beginning advanced study in a chiropractic college. By the time they are qualified for graduation, they have taken a resident course of study and training totalling an average of 4400 sixty minute class hours. This represents four years of college covering a period of nine months each year.

The basic curriculum of chiropractic education is composed of many subjects. Basic science courses include anatomy, physiology, chemistry, pathology, bacteriology, nutrition, hygiene, sanitation, and public health. Clinical courses include physical, clinical, laboratory, and differential diagnosis; gynecology, obstetrics, pediatrics, orthopedics, roentgenology (X-ray), first aid, gerontology, dermatology, toxicology, psychology, principles and practice of chiropractic, spinal analysis, and adjustive techniques. Elective courses are offered in jurisprudence, ethics, and economics. Some schools may offer instruction in kinesiology, meridian therapy, and minor surgery. This comprehensive educational program offers the modern chiropractor a thorough grounding in the basic health sciences and enables him or her to provide the finest quality health care to the widest possible variety of chiropractic patients.

The majority of college faculty hold Doctor of Chiropractic (D.C.) or Ph.D. degrees. The others with Master's degrees are encouraged to seek advanced training in their area of expertise. Many faculty are graduates of the schools in which they teach, conducting courses like technic, roentgenology, and philosophy which are primarily chiropractic in scope. During the past few years, however, colleges have been recruiting professors outside the profession to teach courses like chemistry, clinical nutrition and psychology, and have made efforts to recruit chiropractic faculty from other schools in order to avoid excessive inbreeding of their staffs.

The colleges put more emphasis on anatomy and neurosciences, and devote little attention to drug therapy, surgery, or epidemiology. Many courses required for graduation compare favorably with those taught in medical schools. In areas of special interest such as clinical nutrition and public health, there are more hours of instruction in chiropractic colleges than in most medical schools. Table 5–1 compares graduation requirements for a medical school and a chiropractic college, both located in the eastern United States.

In order to graduate, students must intern about 900 hours in a college operated clinic and pass either of two tests. Those who pass the National Board of Chiropractic Examiners are recognized by most state licensing boards and by almost half of the Basic Science Exam Boards. The Basic Science Board Exam stresses anatomy, physiology, pathology, bacteriology, chemistry, and public health. It is also given to graduates of medical schools and osteopathic colleges.

TABLE 5–1. COMPARISON OF COURSE HOURS REQUIRED FOR GRADUATION

	Medical School	Chiropractic College
Anatomy	296	800
Biology of Disease/ Biometrics/Cell Biology	562	—[1]
Biochemistry	80	160
Endocrinology	40	(80)[2]
General Medicine	460	—
Chiropractic Technique & Philosophy	—	816
Microbiology	103	192
Neurosciences	120	(272)[3]
Obstetrics & Gynecology	220	160
Pathology	123	336
Pediatrics	220	32
Diagnosis	174 (physical)	480
Radiology	(15)[4]	240
Surgery	460	—
Pharmacology	126	—
Psychiatry/Psychology	249	64
Clinical Nutrition	—	96
Community Medicine/ Epidemiology	18	—
Public Health	—	176
Home-Medical Science	160	—
Socio-Medical Science	66	—
Office Procedure & Jurisprudence	—	32
Clinic	—	888
Electives and other required courses	1700 (incl. clinic)	288
Total Hours	5222	5112

[1]Similar course material offered in various departments
[2]Offered in Dept. of Pathology
[3]Offered in Depts. of Anatomy, Diagnosis, and Physiology
[4]Included with Anatomy, Cell Tissue Biology, and Physiology

STATE LAW: PLAYING BY THE RULES AND REGULATIONS

All states and most Canadian provinces allow chiropractors to adjust the spine and related structures such as the arms and legs and many permit the use of drugless adjuncts like massage, hydrotherapy, heat, cold, exercise, acupressure, and nutritional therapy. However, each state has special regulations defining the nature of chiropractic and limiting the kinds of services provided. Some regulations, such as prohibiting the use of drugs and major surgery, were included at the initiative of the chiropractic profession itself. Others, such as limiting the use of X-rays, were passed at the insistence of organized medicine to limit competition.

In New York, for example, the use of chiropractic X-rays is limited to patients over 18 years of age and chiropractors are not allowed to treat cancer, heart trouble, diabetes, or communicable disease. (However, since chiropractors make no claim to treat specific diseases, they are legally permitted to care for patients with any health problem.) A chiropractor in New York State may not take blood tests, but a chiropractor in Nevada can because all methods of diagnosis are permitted by Nevada state law. The use of drugs or surgery is prohibited in every state except Oregon, which allows removal of warts and other "foreign bodies in the superficial structures and the use of antiseptics and local anesthetics in connection herewith." Regulations for soft tissue manipulation vary as well. Massage is permitted in California as long as it is performed in relation to spinal adjustments. Hawaiian law expressly prohibits chiropractors from performing the Hawaiian practice of "lomilomi or massage" as part of their profession. The myriad of state regulations cover even postmortem conditions. If a person dies of a heart attack or an accident in South Dakota, California, or

Tennessee, a chiropractor may legally sign the death certificate, but not if death occurs in Wisconsin, Massachusetts, Arizona, or twenty-one other states.

THE CHIROPRACTOR'S DOMAIN: ADJUSTMENT OR REFERRAL

Even with years of specialized instruction and strict licensing requirements on state and national levels, chiropractors find some still doubt their qualifications. These can be expressed in the following two questions:

> Doesn't a chiropractor treat too wide a range of disease?
>
> Is a chiropractor qualified to recognize diseases which should receive the attention of a medical doctor?

The answer to the first is no. *Chiropractic is not a disease care or symptom care system.* Although practitioners are taught diagnosis in college, symptoms are only guideposts in selecting the proper clinical procedure to eliminate the first cause of dis-ease, nerve interference.

Chiropractors often address the issue of disease treatment by explaining the chiropractic view of the four phases of illness. Phase one is the *production of cause* which may be interference with nerve transmission somewhere between the brain and one or more organs of the body. The second phase is *alteration of function* or the failure of some organ or organs with a resulting upset in the chemical balance of the body. Phase three includes *symptoms, signs, and syndromes* which tell us we are not feeling well. The fourth phase is *actual structural change* involving the pathological degeneration of tissue in the affected body part.

In chiropractic, the *production of cause* is the vertebral

subluxation leading to dis-ease and altered body function. Eventually, illness or disease takes hold revealing itself in *symptoms, signs, and syndromes.* The medical doctor begins work by classifying and naming the effects of body dysfunction, otherwise known as diagnosis. Then he or she applies treatment to these advanced stages of illness.

The chiropractor, on the other hand, does not diagnose symptoms (which implies distinguishing one disease from another), but analyzes a structural condition and decides how to correct it. If a patient has cancer, a heart condition, or any other disease, he or she is a chiropractic case *as long as a vertebral subluxation exists.* This does not imply that a chiropractic case cannot be a medical case as well. Most people come to chiropractors only after their symptoms are severe. When a patient's condition requires allopathic treatment, it is a chiropractor's duty to refer him or her to the appropriate specialist.

The second question regarding the ability of a chiropractor to recognize diseases which should receive medical attention is closely related to the issue of referral. Although they do not receive the same amount of training in symptomatology as medical doctors, the New Zealand study concluded that "the education and training of a registered chiropractor are sufficient to enable him to determine whether there are contraindications to spinal manual therapy in a particular case, and whether the patient should have medical care instead of or as well as chiropractic care."

Many practitioners point out the majority of their patients come to them after traditional medicine has failed and ailments are already thoroughly documented. Ninety-seven percent refer clients to medical doctors and other specialists when they feel the other can be of most help to the patient. Chiropractors do not claim to overly extend *or* limit their areas of expertise. They are bound by professional ethics to hold the welfare of their patients as their highest goal.

QUALITY CONTROL: THE CHIROPRACTIC PROFESSIONAL ORGANIZATIONS

Currently, there are three national organizations whose role is to establish and maintain standards of education, ethics, and professional competency. They also represent the profession before Congress and other government bodies. The larger organizations promote research programs while all three disseminate information to their members and the general public. Many chiropractors are members of more than one professional organization.

The *American Chiropractic Association* (ACA) is the largest of the three. Founded in 1905, the ACA represents the majority of chiropractors in the United States. Its national headquarters is located in Des Moines, Iowa, and there are state and local associations throughout the country. The ACA sponsors professional councils on mental health, neurology, nutrition, physiotherapy, and sports injuries. Their purpose is to develop a chiropractic focus to health related fields and present their findings to the scientific community and the public.

The *International Chiropractors Association* (ICA) was founded by B. J. Palmer in 1926 to represent the profession's conservatives. Located in Washington, D.C., the ICA is composed of chiropractors throughout the United States and many foreign countries, and its Assembly is composed of elected members of each of fifty states. In addition to promoting chiropractic research, professional standards, and lobbying, the ICA—like the ACA—is involved with student recruitment and sponsors an active program of patient and public education.

The *Federation of Straight Chiropractic Organizations* (FSCO) is relatively new and controversial. Founded in 1976 by a group of extremely conservative chiropractors, the FSCO feels the ICA is too close to the liberal philosophy of the ACA and the Council of Chiropractic Education. Despite its small membership—an estimated 600 chiropractors and students by 1980—it has been regarded as a rebel by the other organizations. Made up of a house of delegates from each affiliate, the FSCO endorses a strict code of professional ethics and education of the public and other chiropractors in its philosophy. It also defends the right of graduates of affiliate schools—Sherman and Adio—to practice throughout the country.

Besides the three groups in the United States, professional organizations exist in most countries where chiropractic is officially recognized. The largest include the Canadian Chiropractic Association, the Australian Chiropractors Association, the British Chiropractors Association, and the European Chiropractic Union which is composed of member organizations throughout the continent. You can write to any of these associations at the following addresses for information:

UNITED STATES

American Chiropractic Association
2200 Grand Avenue, Des Moines, Iowa 50312
publishes *The American Chiropractor*

International Chiropractors Association
1901 L Street N.W., Suite 800
Washington, DC 20036
publishes the *International Review of Chiropractic*

Federation of Straight Chiropractic Organizations
1031 Vermont Street, Lawrence, Kansas 66044
publishes *Impulse*

AUSTRALIA

The Australian Chiropractors Association
P.O. Box 19, Bundoora, Victoria 3083

CANADA

The Canadian Chiropractic Association
1900 Bayview Avenue, Toronto, Ontario M4G 3E6

GREAT BRITAIN AND EUROPE

The British Chiropractors Association

The European Chiropractic Union
137 Brighton Road, Sutton, Surrey, England

JAPAN

Japanese Chiropractic Society
9-5-3 Chrome, Kitaaoyama Minato-Ku, Tokyo

NEW ZEALAND

New Zealand Chiropractors Association
P.O. Box 2858, Wellington

SOUTH AFRICA AND ZIMBABWE (RHODESIA)

Chiropractic Association of South Africa
902, Metro Centre, Bree Street, Johannesburg

All chiropractic asssociations have a Code of Ethics and disciplinary procedures for their members. In the United States, each affiliate is similar to its parent organization. It has peer review guidelines implemented when a member's ethics or professional conduct is questioned on either state or local levels. The state operated Division of Professional Licensing Services is equipped to deal with complaints about unethical or incompetent practitioners, be they chiropractors, dentists, optometrists, or medical doctors.

Over the years, the chiropractic profession has reached the highest standards of educational and professional competence. Whether you need help for a physical ailment or preventive care, you can be assured of the services of a trained professional well qualified to perform chiropractic's specialized tasks.

Although practitioners agree on the essential philosophy of their profession—the need to correct nerve interference—the three organizations in the United States highlight the different points of view in chiropractic philosophy and practice. In the following chapter we will examine these varying points of view to see how their different approaches can influence the kind of care we receive.

6

Choosing the Right Chiropractor

According to statistics provided by the Federation of Chiropractic Licensing Boards, there are over 35,000 licensed chiropractors in the United States and Canada. At least one chiropractor can be found in even the smallest hamlet or farm community throughout English and French speaking North America. In rural areas, choice may be limited to the only one in town but those who live in cities and suburbs will want to choose a chiropractor who meets their needs best.

As with any health professional, selection should be a careful and thorough process. After locating the name of a chiropractor, find out his or her standing in the community. Decide whether this person's philosophy of health and disease is compatible with your own and decide if you want the services of a "mixer" or a "straight" practitioner. Find out which techniques will be used in your care. Many want to know the extent of the use of X-rays, and if they are required before care begins. Be sure to understand the financial aspects. Find out if long term contracts are required before the chiropractor will begin giving adjustments. Finally, see how the chiropractor feels about promises of "miracle cures" and if patients are referred to other practitioners when necessary.

FINDING BEFORE CHOOSING: SOURCES

The first logical step in choosing a chiropractor is to find one. This can be done by writing one of the professional organizations listed in Chapter 5, looking in a local newspaper or weekly advertiser, or using the Yellow Pages in a local phone book. It may list chiropractors according to the town or neighborhood in which they practice.

The most reliable way to find one is to ask friends and neighbors. With one American in twenty visiting a chiropractor this year, chances are excellent that you know several patients already. Since the profession is largely dependent on referrals, chiropractors often make a great effort to provide the highest possible level of care. Those who are incompetent or unethical or have difficult personalities will receive little community support. Many encourage patients to bring friends and relatives to witness the examination and adjustment procedure. Some sponsor free lectures to educate the public. Chiropractors feel the more they are observed in practice, the faster myths portraying them as "quacks" and "bone crushers" will dissolve.

If you are a patient already, but expect to move to another community, your present chiropractor can often recommend several others who share the same philosophy and technique you are accustomed to. If you want chiropractic maintenance during a journey, the practitioner may be able to provide a set of your X-rays along with a list of recommended professionals to consult on your trip.

YOUR CHOICE: A MIXER OR A STRAIGHT

Many patients choose a chiropractor for a particular philosophy and range of services rather than for personality or standing in the community. As pointed out in Chapter 3, most chiropractors agree on the basic principles as taught by Daniel David Palmer, but differ on secondary considerations regarding the scope and practice of their profession. While all licensed chiropractors are qualified to locate, analyze, and remove subluxations of the spine, their various attitudes towards health care play a major role in what care we receive. The conflict involves two groups in the profession known as "mixers" and "straights."

A Contrasting View on Health and Disease

The cause of ill health is the root of the basic philosophical difference. Although all chiropractors agree that a healthy nervous system is of primary importance for the maintenance and recovery of health, some early chiropractors did not agree with D. D. Palmer's contention that 95 percent of all disease is caused (directly or indirectly) by spinal subluxations. They believed, as most do today, that mental attitude, environment, heredity, and nutrition play a major role in determining health and resistance to illness. This led them to an interest in other aspects of disease since they regarded vertebral subluxations as just one factor of many. Those who held this view were called "mixers" by D. D. Palmer.

Defenders of Palmer's "straight" approach did not discount the importance of the factors listed above, but pointed out that pollution, poor diet, and an emotional state do greatest damage by causing subluxations which in turn cause nerve interference and ill health. Noting that spinal misalignments are a major threat to the body's ability to adapt to stress, defend itself from germs, and heal itself, they felt the correction of subluxations was their primary goal as specialists in chiropractic. Leave other aspects of health care to other specialists.

The two approaches result in different goals. Straight chiropractors are primarily interested in locating, analyzing, and correcting vertebral subluxations which are held to be the primary cause of dis-ease and dis-order. As long as there is *no interference* to normal functioning, inner wisdom will heal the body as it sees fit. While they agree that many disease states have been known to respond to chiropractic adjustments, straights claim it is an indirect result of the removal of nerve interference rather than a therapeutic procedure as such. Straights place their confidence in the body's ability to "bounce back" after an adjustment alone while their colleagues feel additional techniques should be introduced to help the body attain a normal level of function.

The mixing chiropractors believe that correcting subluxations is only part of the holistic approach to patient care. They believe their role involves diagnosis and treatment of disease by a variety of techniques like blood tests, urinalysis, electrocardiograms, and muscle testing (applied kinesiology) to determine the nature and extent of the complaint. Mixers often apply adjunctive therapies such as acupressure, massage, vitamin therapy, and even hypnosis to provide the widest range of natural services to their patients and see no conflict in offering drugless therapies in addition to chiropractic adjustments.

Diagnosis Versus Analysis

The whole issue of "diagnosis and treatment" of disease is a major source of conflict between the two camps. Mixers use both terms in practice. Straights take pains to use the words "analysis" and "correction."

Mixers point out that the term "diagnosis" has several meanings. One definition states it involves the art of recognizing a disease by the symptoms through examination of body fluids, secretions, and excretions, or by measuring heartbeat, blood pressure, and body temperature. Medical doctors—and most mixers—use them to determine the nature and degree of pathology and then offer the appropriate therapy to relieve it. Another meaning referring to physical diagnosis involves the use of palpatation, inspection, X-ray, or other methods to identify deviations from the normal (such as spinal misalignments). Mixers claim that physical diagnosis is part of chiropractic and, therefore, the term "diagnosis" should be used within the profession.

Although acknowledging the importance of a well rounded scientific background, straights believe diagnosis in the medical sense is beyond the scope of chiropractic except when referring a patient to a medical doctor. Since straight chiropractors from D. D. Palmer onwards have sought to keep chiropractic a separate and distinct healing art from allopathic medicine, they balk at using terms like "diagnosis" which are generally identified with medical practice. They see their role as peforming chiropractic spinal "analysis" meaning "an examination of anything (such as the spinal column) to distinguish its component parts or elements, separately or in relation to the whole." Since a vertebral subluxation cannot be diagnosed in the medical sense, straights feel that the term "analysis" is a far more appropriate word. They argue that if chiropractors claim to diagnose disease, medical science would have a foolproof case for setting standards of chiropractic education, because diagnosis is a medical specialty. Since doctors are trained extensively in diagnosis and symptomatology, chiropractors who want to compete with them should go to medical school and become manipulative therapists. Straights maintain diagnosis is *not* a primary role of the chiropractor, whose task is to locate, analyze, and remove subluxations.

This does not sit well with the liberal mixers who feel chiropractors are more than qualified to diagnose diseases, and refer a patient when it is beyond their expertise.

Treatment Versus Correction

Let's pretend you are in a chiropractor's office complaining of constipation. After assessing your condition, the mixer would outline a detailed program of treatment to alleviate the symptoms and keep them from returning. In addition to chiropractic adjustments—which may or may not continue after symptoms disappeared—your practitioner may recommend periodic enemas, a high fiber diet, and a variety of herbal teas. If blood tests revealed certain deficiencies, a variety of vitamin and mineral supplements taken with filtered water at every meal may be recommended.

After the straight chiropractor determines that you suffer from a vertebral subluxation, a regular series of adjustments to correct the subluxation would be outlined along with a recommended program of preventive chiropractic care to continue long after the disease symptoms disappear. You might be told that the goal was not relief of constipation, but that it would probably disappear when the body's nerve transmission is restored to normal. If you also had a vitamin deficiency, you would probably be referred to a nutritionist because providing dietary advice or nutritional supplements is not within the straight chiropractor's area of expertise.

The words "treatment" and "therapy" imply disease care, so conservative practitioners prefer not to use them. They claim chiropractic was never meant to stimulate or inhibit body functions. The proper term to use is "correction" (as in "correcting a subluxation") which does not imply the treatment or the cure of pathology or disease state.

CHOOSING: THE PROS AND CONS

Extremes of straight and mixer philosophies can be a source of confusion, particularly when it comes to choosing the kind of care we want for ourselves and our families. Despite the tendency to see one side as right and the other side wrong, both aspects of chiropractic have their positive "core qualities" as well as distortions. By sifting through pros and cons, we can see the essence of their contrasts and choose the type of care we feel will meet our needs.

The positive quality of the straight is in abiding respect for the inborn intelligence of the body and a deep confidence in its ability to heal itself. If you complained of asthma, for example, the practitioner would primarily look for a vertebral subluxation and adjust it. Although aware of any contraindication to chiropractic adjustments (such as spinal tumors or a fractured vertebra) and able to recognize situations which could be referred to a different type of practitioner, he or she would locate, analyze, and adjust the subluxation, trusting that once normal nerve transmission was restored, the body would heal itself from the inside out.

On the negative side, the straight does not become involved with therapeutic approaches that may be beneficial to the patient. If you had constipation and demanded immediate relief, enemas would not be recommended because straight chiropractors are not involved in the treatment of disease. Unlike other practitioners of holistic health care, little attention is paid to lifestyle, diet, and environment. Ultraconservatives claim it is not their concern as chiropractors if you are forty pounds overweight, smoke a pack of cigarettes a day, and eat junk food at every meal. This does not mean they don't care. They feel their specialty is analysis and removal of subluxations which will help you deal with these issues as the body's innate intelligence is able to express itself through a nervous system free of interference. Straights maintain that matters of lifestyle, stress management, and nutrition should be referred to other professionals in their own area of expertise. Such an attitude may annoy patients who want their chiropractor to provide them with a broader range of services.

The best quality of mixers is their open mind to new health trends and their interest in integrating several approaches to health in their work. Mixers often possess a sincere desire to remove pain and help the patient overcome disease. "Whatever will help the patient the most" can be the motto of the highminded mixer.

Their negative aspect is not unlike that of some medical doctors: "I can do anything." In offering a wide variety of therapies to "fix up" a patient, the chiropractor takes on the role of a magician with an arsenal of miracle cures. A higher fee may be charged (a concern among critics), and the patient may become dependent on the practitioner's advice for removing symptoms of illness. Such an attitude is a source of conflict and confusion for the chiropractic patient.

However, the controversy has positive aspects and the consumer is the beneficiary. The wide range of philosophical differences within the profession offers a broad spectrum of quality health care for a variety of patient needs. If you want a form of safe and effective drugless therapy for treatment of a particular disorder, you might consult a mixer, who is eminently qualified to treat a wide range of disorders. On the other hand, if you want health care to remove the cause of dis-ease, keep your body free of nerve interference, and indirectly remove symptoms you would tend to seek the care of a straight.

My own experiences over a ten-year period lead me to believe "mixer" and "straight" are arbitrary classifications which do not always reveal the true value of the chiropractor.

My first encounter was with an Illinois chiropractor after I injured my back by carelessly lifting a typewriter. The adjustment was for emergency purposes only. Our intent was to relieve painful symptoms as quickly as possible. When they were removed, I never returned to him again. My second experience was also with a treatment oriented chiropractor who gave me five chiropractic/acupressure sessions during the course of one week. He "fixed me up" by the end of the week as he promised, and symptoms of fatigue and eye inflammation were relieved.

My third experience, in upstate New York, was with a straight chiropractor whom I consulted after injuring my back chopping firewood. He made it clear that his primary task was not to relieve my condition, but to correct subluxations. In addition, he stressed that ongoing maintenance was a key to good health. I continued to see him during the following year for preventive care. My fourth and present chiropractor is a straight whom I see regularly for preventive care. I have always felt healthy, but now I am more resistant to stress and fatigue.

In the preparation of this book, I have interviewed many practitioners and dozens of patients. Although I have a personal preference for straight chiropractors and refer others to my own for care, I enjoy warm personal relations with several "mixers" and refer people to them when I feel the particular chiropractor will meet their needs. I have come to the conclusion that regardless of philosophical belief, overall intent is of far more value to the patient. Is the chiropractor interested in serving or is money the principal factor? Does he or she encourage self reliance or foster dependency? Are adjuncts used to satisfy genuine needs or do they justify a higher fee? Are X-rays used for "appearance value" or are they necessary for proper care? Does the chiropractor reflect good health in personal life, or is it just a theory to talk about? Whether we stand with mixers or straights, answers to the preceding questions will help us select the right chiropractor for our particular needs.

It is important to discover if a practitioner's approach to health is compatible with your needs. Question potential chiropractors regarding their philosophy and techniques. However, since many chiropractors advertise in local telephone directories and newspapers, their advertisements often reveal the kind of practice they maintain. There are no hard and fast rules, but the following key words will reveal the basic orientation:

MIXERS

Holistic approach, adjunctive therapy, treatment (for back pain, headache, nervous tension, etc.), acupressure, massage, physiotherapy, applied kinesiology, traction, nutritional therapy or counseling, vitamin therapy, ACA member

STRAIGHTS

Omit all of the above terms but may include removal of nerve interference, preventive chiropractic care, restoration of nerve function, correction of vertebral subluxations or misalignments, straight chiropractor, family chiroprator, ICA member, FSCO member

Care: Prevention or Crisis

If you prefer health care which removes disease symptoms, many fine chiropractors can satisfy your needs. Learn if they specialize in therapy from advertisements or call and ask if it is featured in their practice.

Some, however, will refuse to accept patients who insist on viewing chiropractic as a form of crisis medicine without drugs. Where such a practioner takes your case, even if you suffer from a disease or other conditions, he or she will make it clear that the goal is not to treat symptoms. Unlike therapy oriented practitioners, these chiropractors emphasize preventive health, and often insist that you return periodically for regular examinations and corrective adjustments if the need exists.

X-Rays: Sometimes, Always, or Never

Most chiropractors take X-rays at one time or another as part of the regular examination. The use of X-rays, however, varies considerably. Some use them rarely, limiting radiation to specific areas of the spinal column, but others frequently use full-spine X-rays which photograph from the base of the skull to below the pelvis to get an idea of how the entire spine is affected by vertebral subluxations.

Although most patients feel uncomfortable about the idea of being X-rayed, an X-ray will determine if any contraindications to chiropractic care exist. For example, a hairline fracture of the second cervical vertebra may escape the scrutiny of a chiropractor during the initial examination. If an adjustment were given, there would be a chance the vertebra would break apart and injure a delicate vein or artery. X-rays also give a better understanding of the nature and extent of the vertebral subluxation, and enable the practitioner to make a more exacting adjustment.

If you have never been to a chiropractor before, or are seeing one as a result of an accident, spinal X-rays are generally a good idea and will lead to better care. If you are concerned about increased radiation risk, ask for smaller X-rays focussing on specific areas of your spine. If it is advised you have follow-up X-rays a month later, be satisfied they are necessary and not just a routine procedure. If you move to another community and plan to see a chiropractor there, ask for your current X-rays. They may not reflect the condition of your spine at the moment, but your next chiropractor will have a better idea of your major problems.

Some practitioners have a "waiver of X-rays" form for patients who refuse them. The waiver, signed by the patient, releases the chiropractor from responsibility if "any untoward effects develop or any further illness or injury develop directly or indirectly" as a result of treatment given without a complete chiropractic examination (to include X-rays, presumably) as recommended. These are used to encourage patients to accept X-rays, but some opt to sign it nevertheless and assume full legal responsibility for their care.

If you are concerned about the dangers of frequent radiation, you may want to select a chiropractor who does not require it as a prerequisite. Also, reject any practitioner advertising free X-rays. Radiation should never be used as a lure.

Techniques: All Safe, All Effective

Since adjustive techniques correct subluxations safely and effectively, selecting a chiropractor who uses a particular style is basically a matter of personal preference. In upstate New York, I went to a chiropractor (Dr. T.) whose technique was very gentle. He believed a light adjustment was just as effective as one involving more force. Some of his adjustments were so gentle one could hardly feel them. Dr. T. had literally hundreds of satisfied patients, but some preferred to visit Dr. L., whose method was more forceful and gave them the feeling that more was being done for them. In reverse, some of Dr. L's patients found Dr. T.'s gentle touch more to their liking.

The Palmer method of adjustment features a dynamic thrust and rapid recoil, while Dr. de Jarnette developed a slower, less dramatic technique. Some chiropractors include light massage as a relaxing adjunct to adjustment. Others may play quiet music to help the patient relax. It is rare to find two chiropractors with identical method and office procedures. Whatever the technique, chiropractic adjustments are all safe, painless, and effective as long as they are administered by a licensed chiropractor.

The final consideration of technique springs from the essential foundation of chiropractic—adjustment by hand. The majority of practitioners adhere to this fundamental concept, but a few use machines to perform spinal corrections. Such devices (which sometimes resemble a drill press) may impress the patient, but most chiropractors believe the safest, most effective way to make adjustments is by hand only.

The Payment Schedule: Know the Cost

Most chiropractors have a flat office fee payable by cash, check, or credit card at the conclusion of each visit. Discounts for ten or twelve adjustments paid in advance may be offered to encourage the patient to return for a predetermined number of visits within an allotted period of time.

The question of payments can be important although some do not feel it is a major factor in choosing a chiropractor.

Besides financial aspects, regularity is important in successful chiropractic care. Advance payment may encourage you to keep appointments and continue adjustments though the initial symptoms disappear.

Before you decide, discuss finances with the practitioner and work out a payment schedule comfortable to both. Remember that restorative chiropractic care is covered by Medicare and Medicaid in many states and most private insurance companies include chiropractic in their health insurance policies. Your chiropractor would know if you are eligible for such insurance, and will provide the appropriate forms to help you make claims.

Rates vary widely, but are usually half the regular office fee of a medical doctor in general practice. The range of care is an important cost factor. A simple adjustment from a straight chiropractor costs between eight and fifteen dollars (1980 prices) and requires about five to ten minutes of office time. On the other hand, one who uses a variety of supplementary therapies would probably spend twenty to forty minutes with the patient and charge $25 or more for a visit.

Other cost factors are determined by the chiropractor as an individual. One, I know, would charge $12 if you wanted to be adjusted immediately, and $6 if you didn't mind waiting in line. Another would charge $8 for an individual visit, and a flat rate of $15 for the entire family, even if it included ten children. It may be difficult to evaluate a chiropractor by the fee, but comparative shopping will help you find chiropractic care at the lowest possible price.

NOTES OF CAUTION

Promises, Promises

Chiropractic is an original approach because it is a health care system rather than a disease care system. It claims that spinal adjustments correct subluxations which help restore the nervous system to greater efficiency, and that as nerve interference is removed, a state of health is more likely to exist. Therefore, it is important to avoid chiropractors who promise complete cures in advertisements or in person, even if they cite cases similar to yours which have responded to chiropractic adjustments.

Contracts

Beware of any chiropractor (or any other practitioner for that matter) who asks you to sign a contract for services. A written agreement is not a customary practice and should be rejected. Very few patients have been victimized by licensed chiropractors, but if a contract is offered as a prerequisite to care, seek legal counsel before you sign, or simply find another chiropractor.

Your Chiropractor and Beyond: Referrals

It is important to find a practitioner (chiropractor or not) who is willing to refer you when another practitioner can do the most good. Over 95 percent of all chiropractors make referrals, so if your doctor does not refer patients—or maligns other practitioners or health care professions—you may want to find someone else. A degree of openmindedness and respect for the basic good intent of other practitioners despite philosophical differences is the mark of a mature and sensitive doctor worthy of your attention.

7

A Visit to a Chiropractor: What to Expect

KENNETH MORRISON, A 32-YEAR-OLD HOUSE painter, appeared to be in satisfactory health. He often complained of neck pain and occasional early morning headaches, however. One of his co-workers suggested that Dr. Roberts, a local chiropractor, might be able to help him. Ken set up an appointment for the following Thursday after work.

When he entered the chiropractor's waiting room, Ken noted with surprise how healthy the other patients looked.

After receiving a warm welcome from the receptionist, he was given a case history to fill out. Although the form was similar to those used by medical doctors, it went into specifics about musculoskeletal complaints and asked him to make note of any fall, sprain, or accident he could recall. Although Ken had a good safety record on the job, he remembered that at 17 he was involved in a minor car accident. His head bumped against the windshield, causing it to shatter. Although he had suffered only a few scratches and a headache, Ken's father took him to the hospital emergency room where he was examined and sent home with a clean bill of health. Until he saw the case history form, Ken hadn't given the accident a second thought.

CONSULTATION AND EXAM

By the time Ken completed the form, Dr. Roberts was ready to see him. The chiropractor's adjusting room looked more like a living room than a clinical office. It was free of the antiseptic odors, sterilizers, and needles often found at a medical doctor's. A large adjusting table stood at the center of the room and a model spine lay on the doctor's desk.

While Ken discussed his case with the chiropractor, he was pleased to discover that Dr. Roberts took a personal interest in him and asked him about himself, not just his symptoms. Even though both knew that others were waiting outside, Dr. Roberts didn't seem hurried, discussing the problem patiently in language Ken could understand. Using the model spine as an example, he showed how vertebrae become misaligned and impinge on spinal nerves. With the aid of a chart depicting the distribution of nerves throughout the body, Dr. Roberts showed how nerve interference in one part of the body can alter the function of an organ or tissue in another part. "Even a childhood fall from a bicycle can cause a spinal misalignment that can impinge a nerve," he said. "You may not feel the effects for a long period of time. I think your car accident fifteen years ago may have been the beginning of your neck problem."

Dr. Roberts' attitude is typical. According to a survey by the University of Utah College of Medicine, chiropractors generated more patient satisfaction than medical doctors. Patients rated them especially high in personality and ability to explain the problem and its care. After the initial exchange of information, both were ready for the examination.

The doctor asked Ken to remove his shirt and lie face down on the adjusting table, which was heavily padded and fitted with a special notch to cradle his head (Figure 7–1). Dr. Roberts then proceeded to examine his back by hand, carefully palpating (examining by touch) each vertebra for any tenderness or bumps. He asked Ken "Does it hurt here?" when he found a tender area, and recorded his findings.

Special attention was paid to the neck (or cervical) region. The second cervical vertebra (or axis) appeared to be out of alignment. The length of Ken's legs was compared (one was 1/4 inch shorter than the other) and the pelvis was found to be slightly askew.

Dr. Roberts then had Ken stand up and bend to the left, the right, forward, and back. Using a plumb line to determine overall spinal alignment, he found that Ken's left shoulder was slightly lower than the right and his head tilted a bit to the right.

After this postural analysis, Ken sat on the table while his skin temperature was measured by a device called a thermeter

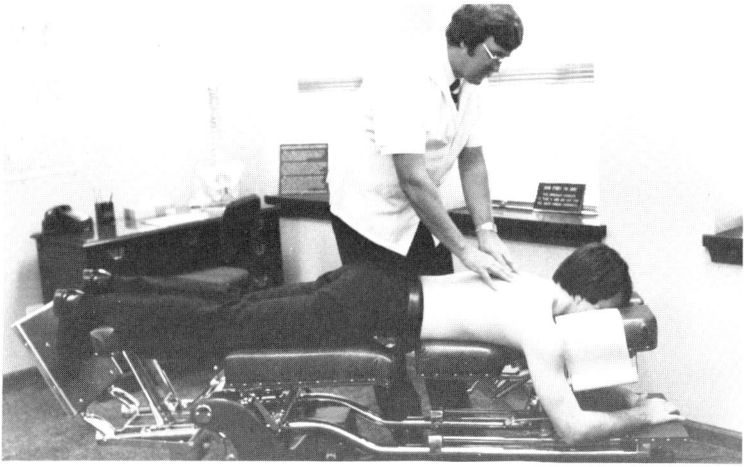

FIGURE 7–1

A chiropractor examining a patient on the popular Zenith® HYLO™ Chiropractic Table. Photo courtesy of Williams Manufacturing, Elgin, Illinois.

(shown in Figure 7–2), a modern successor to the neurocalometer introduced by B. J. Palmer in 1924. Starting from the base of the skull, the doctor carefully moved the two-pronged, hand-held device slowly down the spine, recording differences between one side of the spine and the other. When the temperature is lower on one side, nerve interference may be indicated. In Ken's case, Dr. Roberts found four vertebrae where differences existed and noted their location on Ken's chart. (Other chiropractors sometimes include applied kinesiology—muscle testing—as part of their chiropractic analysis. By testing certain muscles of the body, they can often tell if a related organ or tissue is weak and trace it to a misaligned vertebra.)

Dr. Roberts then brought Ken into the X-ray room and took two pictures of his neck to determine the nature and extent of the suspected misalignment. After analyzing them, earlier findings were confirmed: there was a major subluxation

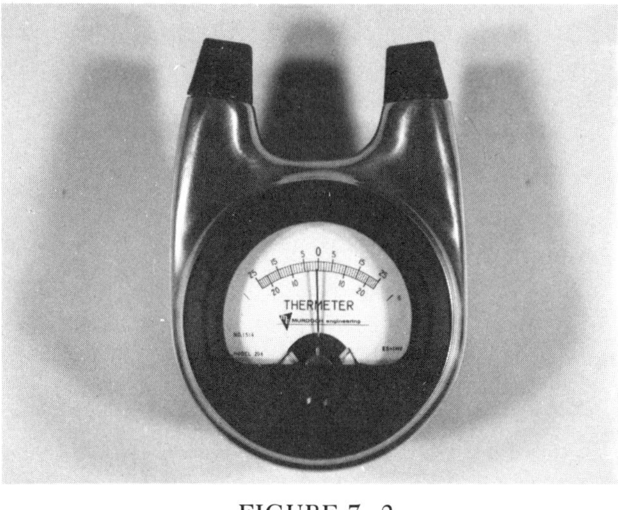

FIGURE 7–2

A thermeter, used to detect heat differentials on either side of the spine. Photo courtesy of Murdoch Engineering.

of the axis or second cervical vertebra which was putting pressure on a nerve. Dr. Roberts said this was contributing to a stiff neck as well as morning headaches, especially when Ken slept on his right side. He also explained that other subluxations further down the spine were attempts to compensate for this major misalignment in the neck and that they could be corrected as well.

A ten week program of adjustments was drawn up which was typical of nonemergency, but chronic, cases such as Ken's: Two adjustments a week for four weeks and one per week thereafter. (Other patients—such as recent accident victims—may begin with five adjustments per week while patients with minor subluxations would start with one.) At the end of the tenth week, Ken's progress would be evaluated and he would probably need preventive maintenance only once a month thereafter. Chiropractors like Dr. Roberts often recommend preventive care long after the original subluxations are corrected. Because chiropractic is based on the body's natural ability to restore and maintain good health, regular chiropractic adjustments are seen as an essential means of keeping the nervous system free from interference and dis-ease.

Ken was pleased that Dr. Roberts's fee would be about half that of his medical doctor and covered by his health insurance plan. After making appointments for future visits, Ken was ready to receive his first spinal adjustment.

THE ADJUSTMENT

Dr. Roberts first took another temperature reading along the spinal column and wrote it in the record book. He then asked Ken to lie down on the table on his stomach, with his head turned to the right. At this point Ken tensed up a little, expecting a great deal of pain from the adjustment, but Dr. Roberts reassured him. Carefully applying light pressure on

Ken's neck just below the right ear, he gave a sudden rapid downward thrust that made an audible "click." He did the same to a point on the upper back (as seen in Figure 7–3) and had Ken, still in a prone position, cross his left leg over the other before he gave the sacrum another rapid thrust. Although he felt a tingling sensation in his head immediately after the adjustment, Ken was surprised to have felt no pain at all. After a few minutes of rest, he got up from the table, stretched, and observed that his neck felt better than it had in years. Dr. Roberts replied that his response was far from unusual. "Your nerve was impinged for over fifteen years," he said. "All we did was remove the interference."

Over the next ten weeks, Ken received a total of fourteen chiropractic adjustments, and began feeling better than he had since high school. He had more energy, felt greater optimism about life, and had an exhilarating absence of neck pain. He wondered why he had put up with it so long.

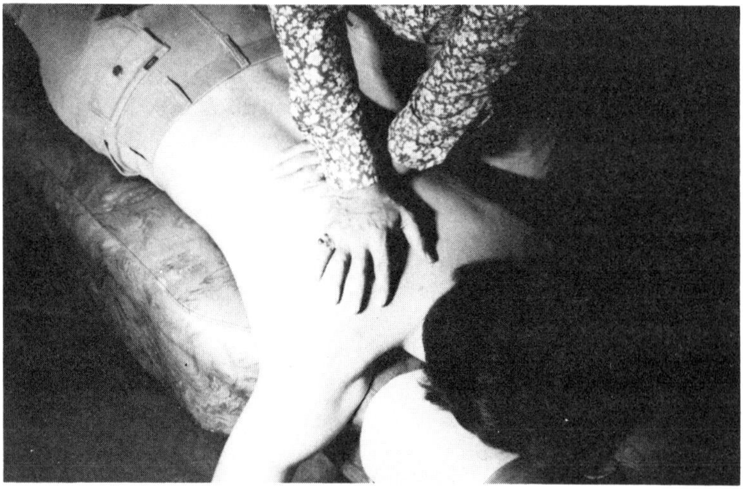

FIGURE 7–3

A patient receiving a chiropractic adjustments. Photo courtesy of Dr. Carl Tompkins.

This experience prompted Ken to ask how often a patient should be adjusted. There was no standard rule to follow, he was told. Schedules for adjustments have been known to vary from twice an hour (usually in an emergency situation where a high fever is present and the patient's life is in danger) to two or three times a week (for a patient with a chronic subluxation). After the initial problem is brought under control, preventive care is scheduled once or twice a month.

Some chiropractors suggest adjustments be discontinued as soon as symptoms disappear, but the majority believe preventive maintenance should involve a long term commitment. Many patients balk at receiving adjustments for years to come, but others feel that continuing maintenance will help preserve health and avoid the pain, disability, and financial cost involved when ill health due to dis-ease occurs.

Dr. Roberts had given Ken a pamphlet by the second visit. It described an exercise program (similar to that in Chapter 10) to help strengthen his spinal muscles and avoid subluxations. An extra firm bed was recommended to replace Ken's old sagging mattress. The doctor also taught him the proper way to lift heavy, bulky objects to reduce the chances of subluxating his spine. Finally, Dr. Roberts encouraged Ken to improve his diet, and suggested several books on nutrition and food preparation. He stressed the better our diets, the less chance we have of subluxating the spine due to toxins and devitalized foods.

Thanks to Dr. Roberts, Ken took a new interest in his health and joined a class in relaxation at the local community college. Through a regular program of preventive care with Dr. Roberts and a personal program of exercise, diet, and stress management, Ken discovered that taking responsibility for his health was exciting and far easier than he had imagined.

Although Ken may be a typical patient and Dr. Roberts a typical chiropractor who confines his practice largely to spinal adjustments alone, the chiropractic profession itself is noted for variety and the ability to provide the kind of care patients want. While some chiropractors rarely use X-rays and make judgments solely on their sense of touch and visual observation, others—who believe that X-rays show many spinal abnormalities which may require special caution—take a series of exposures before they adjust a patient and follow-ups after every few months of treatment.

AN ENVIABLE SAFETY RECORD

Some degree of hazard exists in every technique or occupation, and something may go wrong despite every reasonable precaution whether we speak of chiropractic or any other health system. However, when we compare the percentage of mishaps between chiropractic and medical care, the chiropractor's safety record is an enviable one. Despite the AMA's attacks on the profession as useless, unscientific, and even dangerous, malpractice claims against chiropractors are extremely rare. The high rates of iatrogenic disease, inaccurate diagnosis, and skyrocketing claims for medical malpractice show that the medical profession is hardly in a position to criticize other health care professions for lack of safety or effectiveness.

The respected New Zealand Commission referred to chiropractic as "remarkably safe." Despite its long vendetta against chiropractic, organized medicine has only cited a few documented cases of injury out of millions of adjustments given each year. Most of these were due to underlying pathologies like tumors and artery conditions which the chiropractor was not able to recognize.

Isolated cases of accident and poor judgment have occurred. One case of malpractice appeared years ago when a chiropractor promised to cure a little girl of cancer, convincing her parents not to send her to a medical doctor for treatment. After the child died, the chiropractor was convicted of second-degree murder. With rare exceptions such as this, practitioners will not claim to cure any disease, let alone a life threatening illness like cancer. They are trained to distinguish a chiropractic case from a medical one, and to refer the latter to the proper specialist for treatment.

Another question involves the chiropractor's ability to suggest that patients discontinue taking medication. Unlike medical doctors, chiropractors do not have extensive training in pharmacology and drug therapy because they do not use medication in their practice. What they do know in these areas is often self taught. For this reason there have been isolated cases of practitioners recommending patients to discontinue certain medications with unfortunate results. *Pennsylvania Medicine* cited one which was published in *Consumer Reports:* "Under chiropractic care, an elderly woman with high blood pressure was advised to stop medication. Her blood pressure rose sharply and after a month she suffered a stroke."

Although such a case is rare, it illustrates that chiropractors are not in the position to recommend that patients discontinue medication. Very often, as adjustments restore proper nerve transmission and the body's functions return to normal, the patient needs less and less medication. However, responsible chiropractors leave such a decision to the patient and recommend their medical doctor be consulted when such a step is contemplated.

As mentioned earlier, adjustments performed by a licensed chiropractor provide maximum results with minimum risk. However, there is a danger with "chiropractic-type" manipulation performed by unqualified people. Although osteopaths, physiotherapists, and some medical doctors receive partial instruction in the art of spinal manipulation, they have not received extensive training in chiropractic adjusting techniques, which only a chiropractor is qualified—and licensed—to perform. The Commission of Inquiry on Chiropractic addressed this issue, concluding that "chiropractors are the only health practitioners who are necessarily equipped by their education and training to carry out spinal manual therapy (chiropractic adjustments)" and that "the responsibility for spinal manual therapy training, because of its specialized nature, should lie with the chiropractic profession."

Part 2

BEYOND SPINAL ADJUSTMENTS: CONSTRUCTIVE SURVIVAL VALUES

8

Healthy Intentions

B. J. PALMER TAUGHT AN IMPORTANT CONCEPT called *survival values* as an integral part of chiropractic philosophy. Each of these values, in mathematical terms, is a *unit of adaptational success* of the body to adapt to its environment, permitting the state we call health. Palmer believed that chiropractic adjustments were a primary factor in promoting what he called "constructive survival values" because they enable the body to respond and adapt more easily to its environment by restoring the integrity of the nervous system. On the other hand, vertebral subluxations lead to "destructive survival values" which open the door to dis-ease and ill health.

Besides chiropractic technique, there are aspects of health which can enhance or limit the benefits of chiropractic care. Some believe that as long as they receive regular adjustments they will remain healthy no matter how they abuse their bodies, such as the man who smokes two packs of cigarettes a day for thirty years. Despite the fact he may receive chiropractic adjustments every week, harmful chemical effects from cigarettes may increase the likelihood of subluxation and dis-order.

This and the following chapters explore ways to take more responsibility for our well-being. Chiropractors recommend that a commitment to healthy intentions and relaxation, a wholesome, nutritious diet, and a program of regular exercise will enhance the effectiveness of chiropractic care and help us achieve constructive survival values throughout our lives.

TIPPING THE SCALE FROM NEGATIVE TO POSITIVE

In the following case history, we will compare the positive lifestyle factors (P) and the negative factors (N). See how the two balance out in the life of Suzanne C., a chiropractic patient from California.

The Case of Suzanne C.

Suzanne C. is an executive who enjoys her work at a public relations firm (P) in downtown Los Angeles (N). After a good night's rest (P) she goes jogging with her husband (P) and devotes fifteen minutes to meditation and relaxation (P). She eats a good breakfast of whole grain cereal, fresh fruit, and yogurt (P), kisses and hugs her husband, Tom, goodbye (P), and drives to work on a crowded, slow-moving freeway (N).

Upon entering the office, she learns her company is about to lose an important account (N) and she has been asked to convince the client to stay. After a flurry of tense conferences with her boss (N) and several frustrating phone calls (N) to arrange a meeting with her client, the two women finally agree to meet that evening for dinner. Suzanne manages to take a fifteen minute break to do some stretching exercises (P) while her secretary makes the restaurant reservations.

Leaving work early, Suzanne decides to walk (P) along a quiet route through the park (P) to her chiropractor's office for her regular biweekly adjustment (P). Although feeling some anxiety about the meeting (N), Suzanne believes she can persuade the client not to leave (P).

They meet in a quiet restaurant with relaxed surroundings (P). Suzanne orders a light meal with one glass of wine (P). Despite lingering fears of losing the account (N) her sense of humor puts both Suzanne and her client at ease (P). The meeting goes well, and although no final decision is reached, the client agrees to seriously review her company's wish to seek another agency (P).

Suzanne returns home late that night (N), but is greeted with a warm hug by her husband (P). After Suzanne and Tom share the day's events (P)—he also had a busy day at work—they give each other a relaxing massage (P) before going to bed.

Suzanne's day was not without negative factors: the traffic jam, inner-city pollution, a crisis at work, and anxiety. However, because she also had positive things working for her that day—such as a good diet, physical affection from her husband, regular exercise, relaxation, a sense of humor, and a chiropractic adjustment—she was able to transform negative challenges into opportunities leading to constructive survival values. When figured on a mathematical scale, Suzanne finished her day with a net gain in survival value which had a positive effect on her well-being.

Although under the care of a chiropractor for years, Suzanne knows adjustments are primarily for preventive maintenance and not intended as a "fix" for back strain or headache. Her chiropractor is concerned with a total person, not just a spine, so it was suggested at the very first visit that Suzanne take responsibility for her health to complement the advantages of regular chiropractic care.

Most chiropractors recommend some kind of program which will help achieve constructive survival values in life and the state of positive wellness we all deserve. The following approach to constructive survival values is just one program that can be put into practice.

Step 1: Becoming Aware of the Power of Intent

Paul W., a successful accountant, has just been told by his physician that he has an ulcer. In addition to being afraid, Paul resents being ill and feels like a victim. With a wife and two small children to support, bills to pay, and a job which requires his full attention, an ulcer was the last thing he wanted to deal with.

Most of us don't suffer from ulcers like Paul, but we often feel angry, victimized, and resentful when we become sick. After a lifetime of conditioning by our parents, the media, and the medical profession, we see disease as a result of "germs" or "bad luck," not as a natural result of our inner disharmony or irresponsibility regarding our health.

A genuine desire to be well—also known as "healthy intentions"—is a major ingredient in constructive survival values which B. J. Palmer taught years ago. They are inner attitudes which promote and enhance health in obedience to our intuitive faculties which tell us (often very subtly) how our body's wisdom needs to function without physical or emotional interference. According to Carl Simonton and Stephanie Matthews-Simonton in their important book for cancer patients, *Getting Well Again:* "The unconscious mind contains priceless resources that can be mobilized for personal growth and healing. Indeed, throughout the history of psychological study, theoreticians have proposed the existence of a 'center' in the psyche that directs, regulates, and influences the course of an individual's life."

While chiropractic care helps us become more responsive to inner wisdom, chiropractors recommend we make an effort to be open to intuitive feelings about physical and psychological needs, then use common sense to do what is necessary to fulfill them.

Step 2: Working with the Pleasure Principle

Good health is supposed to be among everyone's goals in life. It is difficult to believe part of us derives pleasure from not being healthy. Sympathy, love, attention from family and friends, time off from work or school, reduced demands on our time, the avoidance of unpleasant responsibilities, getting back at someone else, and other "benefits" of illness often give us a great deal of pleasure. In a society where people are rewarded for being ill (how many of us are given days off from work with pay because we are well?), our subconscious negative intentionality is a difficult habit to transform.

Let's return to Paul W. Although he wasn't aware at the time of diagnosis, Paul had several subsconscious reasons for being sick. In the first place, he was jealous of his wife, who could stay home all day and be closer to the children while he often worked overtime. Paul felt his wife didn't appreciate him enough, only seeing him as a strong man she could depend on (of course, Paul had his part in promoting that image). He disliked his job and resented the boss for making so many demands on his time, especially during tax season. He wasn't sure about his future career and yearned to take a few weeks off in the country to think things over.

Since Paul's wife was a chiropractic patient (for lower back pains), she suggested that her practitioner might help Paul's ulcer. He was soon receiving several adjustments a week which brought him some relief. However, Paul often showed up late for appointments and sometimes forgot them altogether. His chiropractor felt there were hidden factors aside from vertebral subluxations which influenced Paul's ulcer. In a few minutes of conversation during the next visit, the doctor learned of his frustration with his job and the feeling he wasn't really appreciated at home. It was suggested that Paul share his feelings with someone who might help him come to terms with his problems.

With the short-term aid of a therapist, Paul soon discovered his illness satisfied a number of basic needs in his life:

1. He could spend more time at home and enjoy the status his wife had with their children.
2. He was able to receive the sympathy and attention he didn't get from his wife when feeling healthy and "independent."
3. He was able to punish his boss by not being available in the office during a critical period.
4. He was able to give himself some time to relax and think about his future.

Paul was able to work through some of the issues which contributed to his illness. He learned how to express his vulnerable side at home which led to a more intimate relationship with his wife. He was able to restructure his time in the office so that some of the work could be done at home nearer his children. Paul learned to relate better to his boss and relax more on the job. Later, he asked for a transfer to work in an area more interesting to him. Within a month after the initial visit to the counselor, symptoms slowly began to disappear. He was able to "hold" chiropractic adjustments for a longer period of time. His diet began to improve as well, and Paul learned to eat more slowly and enjoy his meals. By becoming aware of his negative intentionality toward health, stressful areas in his life were identified and transformed before a health problem could occur in the future.

Unlike Paul, we can discover our negative intent towards health without getting sick or seeking professional counseling. In their book *Getting Well Again*, the authors suggest making a list of five benefits we get from being sick, especially from a major illness. After the list is made, review it and consider what underlying needs were met. Finally, identify the rules or beliefs which limit us from meeting those needs when we are well. As an illustration, the authors speak of tension:

> Ask yourself if you have been unable to allow yourself periods of relief from tension. What personal beliefs stop you from giving yourself this freedom without needing an illness for justification? . . . Once you begin to become aware of your internal rules and are able to see alternate ways of viewing situations, you are on the road to a healthier life.

Table 8–1, a "habits list" for chiropractic patients, is one way to see how we look at health. It can help us pinpoint our positive feelings and also those areas in our lives which need our attention. Complete the following table. After you are done, ask why you responded as you did. Do your answers reflect a positive statement towards life? Do they say "no" to life? What are some underlying reasons behind the "yes" or the "no"?

The first nine categories—if experienced daily or several times a week—generally reveal feelings of positive intent toward health as does a chiropractic adjustment at least once a month. The latter ten tend to reflect unresolved issues and a possible negative intent. When we discover a negative habit or situation, ask if it is a "pseudosolution" to fulfill certain real needs. For example, does overeating serve as a pseudosolution for other forms of pleasure such as sharing physical affection with another? Does it help to avoid feelings of sadness or anxiety? After finding the truth, seek out positive alternatives to satisfy these needs which will not be stressful to our health.

Step 3: Managing Stress— For Every Pull, Give a Push

Stress is a normal part of life according to Hans Selye, author of *Stress Without Distress*. It is not just nervous tension,

TABLE 8–1. A HABITS LIST

	Once a month or less	Few times a month	Few times a week or daily
1. Engage in sports, jogging, calasthenics, dancing, etc.			
2. Walk 1/2 mile or more			
3. Go out socially			
4. Meditate or pray			
5. Have a period of quiet unthinking relaxation			
6. Have enough sleep			
7. Feel joyous or at peace			
8. Engage in pleasurable sexual activity			
9. Give/receive physical affection			
10. Feel anxious, fearful, or under pressure			
11. Eat too much			
12. Smoke cigarettes			
13. Feel depressed			
14. Feel physical pain			
15. Be exhausted from work			
16. Take mind altering drugs			
17. Feel resentful			
18. Drink enough alcohol to get high			
19. Drink 2 or more cups of coffee a day			

but the body's response to any demand made on it. A family argument or a pleasurable experience like watching a sunset can produce it. Although we would be dead without any stress, Selye points out our ability to adapt to it determines our level of health. Unadaptability leads to *distress* which is linked to a wide range of health problems like hypertension, migraine headaches, heart disease, ulcers, and even cancer.

Chiropractors are aware that stress can cause vertebral subluxations. While regular adjustments will correct the displacements, we can prevent their frequent occurrence by positive use of stress in our lives.

Professionals from various health fields have suggested a number of ways to deal with tension: going for a walk or run, enjoying music, participating in a sport or hobby, reading a book, or working in a garden. Other approaches may be less conventional, but equally effective. Norman Cousins, in his book *Anatomy of an Illness*, told how ten minutes of belly laughter at frequent intervals (he saw Marx Brothers movies and old "Candid Camera" television shows) helped him overcome a life-threatening disease. Humor shouldn't be used as a total escape from life, but integrating "laugh therapy" into each day can relieve tension. B. J. Palmer recognized its value. The following message was painted over the men's urinal in one of the washrooms at the Palmer School of Chiropractic: "Lesson number nine: Don't take yourself too damn seriously."

Another enjoyable way of dealing with daily tension is "hug therapy." Dr. David Bresler of the UCLA Pain Control Unit in Los Angeles prescribes a minimum of four hugs a day for men and women to relieve everyday nervous tension. (A list of books regarding stress management and relaxation can be found in the list of references.)

Step 4: Progressive Relaxation— Tense Up and Let Go

A simple, effective exercise which releases stress involves a selective tensing up and relaxing of voluntary muscles of the body. Not measured by scientific instruments until recently, the benefits of this exercise include a decrease in muscle tension (which can reduce the possibility of vertebral subluxations), heartbeat, oxygen consumption, blood pressure, and respiratory rate. Different methods were introduced by Dr. Herbert Benson in his bestseller *The Relaxation Response* and the Simonton book *Getting Well Again*. A chiropractor I met in Florida suggested the following technique which can be practiced almost anywhere. The best time is before a meal (especially breakfast), but it can be done at any time we are under stress.

1. First, tense the muscles in your face. Hold this tension for a few seconds, then completely relax.
2. Now move down to your neck. Tense the muscles, then completely relax.
3. Repeat this in different sections of the body. Work down through the shoulders, arms, hands, chest, stomach, buttocks, legs, and feet. By the time you reach your feet, a total, relaxed state will result.
4. As a variation, all the muscles of the body can be tensed, then relaxed at the same time, or a particular muscle can be tensed, relaxed, and gently massaged.
5. As the tension is released, let your breath out accompanied with a long "aaahh" or a sigh. This will assist in getting in touch with your deeper feelings and will help release them.
6. Quiet, deep breathing can follow this exercise. Give more attention to any parts of the body which require additional relaxation.

Step 5: Breathe Tension Away

Indian yogis have known the secret of deep rhythmic breathing for thousands of years. It is now recognized by medical doctors as an effective way to improve circulation, decrease heartbeat, lower blood pressure, and reduce muscle tension. It can be enjoyed with a minimum of training. Considered to be a complete relaxation technique by itself, deep breathing can also serve as a foundation for several aspects of meditation like creative visualization, concentration, prayer, receptivity, and the act of sending good feelings to others.

Find a quiet place where you can maintain a straight back comfortably (to avoid tension and vertebral subluxation) and be in a relatively unpolluted environment. Sit in a chair, cross-legged on a mat on the floor, or anywhere else, even in an automobile. Although divided into three basic phases, each inhalation and each exhalation should be one gradual, easy movement.

1. Close your eyes. Inhale gradually through the nostrils, first filling the diaphragm area by exerting a gentle pressure on the abdomen. Do this to the count of four.
2. Gradually fill the middle part of the lungs. Gently push out the lower ribs, breastbone, and chest. Continue the count from four to eight.
3. Fill the higher part of the lungs. Lift the chest slightly for another slow count of four until a count of twelve is reached.
4. Hold this inhalation for three seconds.
5. Gradually exhale to the count of twelve, reversing the order of the inhalation: the upper chest first, then the middle, and finally the diaphragm.

This exercise should be repeated three times at first. Increase the number of repetitions every few days until you reach twelve. There should be no sense of strain either in breathing or during the pauses. Steady rhythm rather than length of time is the aim. The respiratory muscles should relax with every exhalation. Letting go of this tension can then diffuse to all other parts of the body, resulting in a state of general relaxation.

Step 6: Creative Meditation— Communion with Innate

Meditation is not only for yogis and Christian mystics. It can be enjoyed by anyone wishing to get in touch with their own inner wisdom. According to early teachings, the meaning of meditation is to "bring to the center." In chiropractic terms this means the core where our innate intelligence resides. Like the previous two relaxation techniques, recent studies have found that meditation can reduce blood pressure, heartbeat, oxygen intake, and respiratory rate. Some chiropractors believe meditation can prevent subluxations caused by nervous tension and increase the period of time we can hold a chiropractic adjustment. There are dozens of meditation techniques. Most of them share at least four basic elements:

1. Quiet surroundings
2. A comfortable position
3. An object or concept to focus upon
4. A receptive attitude

When I was in India, my chiropractor recommended meditating ten minutes each day to enhance the benefits of the adjustments and acupressure treatments I received. He suggested the following ritual to relax my body, quiet my mind, and put me in touch with innate intelligence, which B. J. Palmer affectionately referred to as "the fellow within."

1. Find a comfortable place where you can be quiet and alone for a short time each day.
2. Select a comfortable position. The chiropractor suggested I use a cushioned, straight-backed chair. Others like to sit cross-legged on a mat, or lie down on their backs on a cushion or thick carpet. The greatest risk of lying down, however, is falling asleep.

3. Those who meditate with their eyes open should select something simple to focus on, like a candle, a flower, a religious symbol or other beautiful object. This will keep your mind from wandering. If you keep your eyes closed, try to visualize a field of white light.

4. Begin breathing slowly and deeply, becoming aware of each breath as it enters and leaves your body. Each time your mind wanders or is distracted, bring it back to the easy, natural rhythm of your breathing. If you have trouble concentrating, count each inhalation and exhalation up to ten. Then start over again.

5. As you relax physically, various thoughts and feelings come and go. They shouldn't be repressed. Calmly observing them may cause them to lose intensity.

6. Gradually intuit and then visualize a particular quality as the keynote of your day: patience, strength, compassion, understanding. Express your desire to the "friend within" to help make this virtue an integral part of your life during the day, either in silence or aloud. "I want to" (or "I pray to") "be patient at work and feel my inner strength throughout the day." Repeat this desire slowly several times. Express other desires you want to reflect during the day. These expressions help you adapt to the outer environment from a place of inner stability and poise.

7. After expressing your keynote quality, relax and be receptive once more. Continue breathing deeply for at least three minutes. Feel this core quality as living inside your body, near the heart.

8. This phase may be followed by repeating a sound, known in India as a *mantra*. You may choose to repeat the Sanskrit word *OM*, the most sacred word in the

Hindu religion, three times slowly (one time per slow exhalation). You can also use the word *Shanti* (Sanskrit for peace); an English word like Peace, One, Harmony, Right Thought, Right Action, or a complete phrase like "Thy Will Be Done."

9. Spend another minute or so in a receptive state. End your meditation gradually and in silence.

Practice this form of simple meditation for ten minutes at first. If it feels comfortable, work up to fifteen or twenty minutes. For best results, try to experience this "quiet time" at least once a day at a regular time and place. If you can't devote ten minutes a day, try two minutes or five minutes. Meditation should be a pleasure and not a drudge.

There are many other aspects of healthy intentions like choosing an enjoyable career, learning to enjoy work, taking up a hobby, learning how to express feelings, learning how to confront others in a spirit of love without holding a grudge, and learning how to create pleasure in daily life (taking time for a walk, visiting good friends, treating yourself to a bubble bath, or giving yourself the vacation or special gift you've always wanted). Although these methods and enjoyments may appear frivolous at first glance, they reflect a deeper intent to avoid tension, disharmony, and fatigue and create constructive survival values in our lives.

Healthy intentions are an integral part of the chiropractic process because they lead us to seek preventive chiropractic care. By consciously working to achieve constructive survival values in daily life, we help our chiropractor keep us free from vertebral subluxations: a primary cause of dis-ease. We actively participate in our well-being by recognizing and transforming destructive beliefs and unhealthy practices which create subluxations and inhibit our natural healing process into attitudes and practices which help us enjoy life to the fullest.

9

Eating for Life and Spine

DIET HAS BEEN OF INCREASING CONCERN among health care professionals, but chiropractic's focus on nutrition is unique. While agreeing that poor diet can lead to ill health, chiropractors focus on a frequently unrecognized aspect: poor dietary habits can open the door to subluxation and dis-ease *first* which, in turn, lead to a wide variety of degenerative diseases like atherosclerosis, arthritis, and diabetes later in life.

For this reason, good nutrition has always been an important concern of chiropractic. In the early 1900's several of the training colleges taught nutrition and dietetics as part of their regular curriculum, while most other colleges—and medical schools in particular—felt nutrition was of minor importance. This attitude among medical schools has changed during the last ten years or so, but the chiropractor's training in clinical nutrition far surpasses that of the average medical student today.

One of the first chiropractic books to discuss diet and nutrition was *The Chiropractic Textbook* by R.W. Stephenson, D.C. Although concern about artificial food additives and environmental pollution did not capture the public interest until recently, Dr. Stephenson addressed these issues nearly sixty years ago: "Anything made or prepared artificially and then introduced into the body, against which Innate rebels, is a poison. Foods, air, or water when they have been 'doctored' are poisons."

B. J. Palmer also took a strong interest in nutrition but warned that prescribing specific diets was contrary to the basic philosophy of chiropractic. He believed each person had unique dietary needs and could intuitively choose the needed foods if given the chance (provided that nerve supply was unobstructed by subluxations). He claimed the educated intelligence of the chiropractor could not presume to know what kind of diet the patient's innate intelligence required for the body's optimum health.

Although Palmer's point is well taken, other chiropractors believe that nutritional counseling is part of their job. One pointed out that since nutritional guidance is not offered by most health practitioners, chiropractors have a responsibility to fill a vital need which is often ignored. A diet free of poisons and rich in essential nutrients can help prevent the onset of vertebral subluxations and keep patients free of dis-ease.

It is difficult to find two chiropractors who completely agree on what an optimum diet should be. There is a tendency to avoid extremes, working with each individual to formulate a balance compatible with his or her needs. These diets are, generally, low in fat, refined sugar, and other processed foods, but provide sufficient vitamins, minerals, proteins, and other food elements essential for good health. Some practitioners also advise supplements of commercial vitamin and mineral preparations.

EATING FOR HEALTH

The first step a chiropractor may take in creating a dietary program is a health history. Special attention would be given to any nutrition related disorders such as constipation, diabetes, or high blood pressure as well as problems of overweight, underweight, skin disorders, or insomnia. The patient would be asked about lifestyle and physical activity: "Do you sit at a desk all day long? Do you exercise daily? How far do you walk to the supermarket? Do you perform housework or other regular physical tasks?"

The chiropractor may suggest the patient prepare a nutritional diary in order to find the amount and variety of foods he or she consumes during the week. There is no standard form for such a diary, but Eleanor Gilpatrick, Ph.D., tells students taking her *For Ecology of Health* course at Hunter College in New York City to set up a weekly chart. Her instructions are in Table 9–1.

To provide more effective nutritional guidance, some chiropractors want to learn about their patients' deeper attitudes regarding certain foods. You may be asked to fill out a questionnaire on which you list the foods you consume, how often you consume them, how you feel about your food intake, and which foods you try to include or avoid in your daily diet.

Good nutrition is our personal responsibility, and practitioners feel they need to be aware of the patient's underlying intent towards food and health before a particular nutritional program that will work can be recommended.

A primary concern among chiropractors is the adulterated and unhealthy foods that make up the basic diet of the majority of people living in industrialized countries such as ours. Such food can produce vertebal subluxations, help us put on weight, stimulate us when we are tired, and make us numb when we are tense. Chiropractors warn that when we lose touch with our body's innate intelligence, we are unable to give it what it really needs.

Many people select "empty calorie" foods like pastry, sugary drinks, and candy which are high in calories yet low in essential vitamins and minerals. Consumption of these in place of foods like whole grains, fruits, vegetables, and legumes are of concern to nutritionists who observe that many of us become fat and undernourished at the same time.

TABLE 9–1

Fill in the food you eat each day. Try to list what you eat as soon as you eat it. This includes breakfast, lunch, dinner, between meal snacks, coffee breaks, bedtime snacks, etc. Include coffee, tea, water, alcoholic beverages, candy, and "munchies" in front of the TV set. List everything, even what you may not be too happy about. Reprinted courtesy of Dr. Eleanor Gilpatrick.

Day	Breakfast	Between Meals	Lunch	Between Meals	Dinner	Between Meals
Wed.						
Thur.						
Fri.						
Sat.						
Sun.						
Mon.						
Tues.						

HEALTH SURVEY

INTAKE

Check the items that best describe your *current* intake and attitudes.

	Frequency			Attitude	
	Never or Rarely	Few Times Per Month	Several Times Per Week or Daily	Try to Avoid	Try to Include
1. Meat	___	___	___	___	___
2. Fish, fowl	___	___	___	___	___
3. Eggs	___	___	___	___	___
4. Milk, cheese, yogurt	___	___	___	___	___
5. Whole grains	___	___	___	___	___
6. Peas, beans, lentils	___	___	___	___	___
7. Nuts, seeds	___	___	___	___	___
8. Fresh or dried fruit	___	___	___	___	___
9. Cooked fruits, vegetables	___	___	___	___	___
10. Raw vegetables	___	___	___	___	___
11. Bran, roughage	___	___	___	___	___
12. Vitamin supplements	___	___	___	___	___
13. Mineral supplements	___	___	___	___	___
14. Protein supplements	___	___	___	___	___
15. Water	___	___	___	___	___
16. Sugar as additive, any form	___	___	___	___	___
17. Coffee, caffeine, tea, other caffeine drinks	___	___	___	___	___
18. Alcohol	___	___	___	___	___
19. Aspirin and other non-prescription medicine(s)	___	___	___	___	___
20. Refined grains, starches	___	___	___	___	___
21. Other processed foods	___	___	___	___	___
22. Salt as additive	___	___	___	___	___
23. Food coloring	___	___	___	___	___

Table 9–1 (continued)

	Frequency: Never or Rarely	Frequency: Few Times Per Month	Frequency: Several Times Per Week or Daily	Attitude: Try to Avoid	Attitude: Try to Include
24. Food preservatives	___	___	___	___	___
25. Saturated, hydrogenated fats, oils	___	___	___	___	___
26. Polyunsaturated fats	___	___	___	___	___
27. Prescription medicine(s): (Fill in which)					
______	___	___	___	___	___
______	___	___	___	___	___
28. Mind altering drugs: (Fill in which)					
______	___	___	___	___	___
______	___	___	___	___	___

29. Do you currently smoke? Check one below:
Never ______ Rarely ______ About half pack per day ______
About pack per day ______ More than pack per day ______

FEELINGS ABOUT INTAKE:

	Good and Healthful	Fairly Healthful	Not Good, and Would Like Help	Not Good, and Don't Want Help
1. My food intake is:	___	___	___	___
2. My liquid intake is:	___	___	___	___
3. My food supplement intake:	___	___	___	___
4. My alcohol intake is:	___	___	___	___
5. My use of medications is:	___	___	___	___
6. My use of drugs is:	___	___	___	___
7. My use of tobacco is:	___	___	___	___
8. My overall diet is:	___	___	___	___
9. Conditions under which I eat, when I eat, and the time I give to it are:	___	___	___	___

Nearly one third of the population is considered "obese" by the United States government. This is a concern among chiropractors. Normally, the spine is held in place by ligaments and muscles which efficiently support it. Overweight disturbs the spine's proper muscle tone because the abdomen needs more support. As a result, subluxations occur. Any extra baggage subjects the entire body to unnecessary stress and strain that can limit our ability to enjoy a long, healthy life.

For these reasons, the American Chiropractic Association Council on Nutrition has prepared a "Ten Most Unwanted List." These foods and other items are consumed in large quantities by the majority of Americans and should be replaced by those that are healthier.

1. White refined sugar and candy
2. Alcoholic beverages
3. Coffee
4. Cola beverages or artificially colored drinks
5. Artificially flavored products with too many preservatives added
6. "Junk foods" and snacks
7. White flour products
8. Hot dogs and some fast-food outlet items
9. Tobacco
10. Prepared foods, such as TV dinners and numerous other "quick" convenience foods.

TOWARD A NATIONAL FOOD POLICY

Aware of the need for improved dietary guidelines, the chiropractic profession took great interest in the establishment of the Senate Select Committee on Nutrition and Human Needs chaired by Senator George S. McGovern of South Dakota. Known as the McGovern Committee, it sponsored extensive hearings in Washington from 1969–1977 to help determine dietary guidelines for the United States which were conducive to sound nutrition and good health. The following recommendations were issued in February 1977 under the title *Dietary Goals for the United States:*

1. Increase consumption of fruits and vegetables and whole grains.
2. Decrease consumption of (red) meat and increase consumption of poultry and fish.
3. Decrease consumption of foods high in fat and partially substitute polyunsaturated fat for saturated fat.
4. Substitute nonfat milk for whole milk.
5. Decrease consumption of butterfat, eggs, and other high cholesterol sources.
6. Decrease consumption of sugar and foods high in sugar content.
7. Decrease consumption of salt and foods high in salt content.

The recommendations were regarded as conservative by many nutritionists and health experts, but representatives of the meat, egg, sugar, dairy, and salt industries which could not benefit from the recommendations condemned them as radical and irresponsible. Conservative sectors of the medical profession like the AMA joined with industry. The Senate committee was forced to issue a revised set of dietary guidelines that would be more in accord with industry needs. As a result, the call to "eat less meat" was replaced with the innocuous "eat less saturated fat" while the specific original recommendations were paraphrased with such vague admonitions as "eat a variety of foods," "avoid too much fat," "eat foods with adequate starch and fiber," and "avoid too much sugar."

Whether we follow the guidelines of the McGovern Committee or any other set of recommendations, it is important our dietary goals provide good nutrition and a minimum of toxins. Although ideas will differ according to personal taste, location, ethnic background, and our general level of activity, there are guidelines that can be followed by everyone.

QUALITY, NOT QUANTITY

Although most chiropractors know more about nutrition than the average medical doctor, Dr. Michael C. is one of a rare breed of chiropractors who has taken a postgraduate course in nutrition at a major state university. As a progressive health educator in addition to a licensed chiropractor, Dr. C. sees strong parallels between chiropractic and a healthy diet:

> Chiropractic works with the living forces of nature. Wholesome, fresh and pure foods are the best sources of this vital force, especially when eaten in their natural state. This is why I recommend a diet that includes a variety of whole grains, raw seeds and nuts, sprouts, fresh fruits and vegetables—the purest and most vital foods a person can eat. With a minimum of imagination and a few good cookbooks you can use these foods in hundreds of fantastic recipes that will save you money and be good to your body.
>
> Meat? You don't need it. A well selected diet without meat can provide more than enough of your protein requirements. But if you really want meat, fish and poultry are lower in fat than red meat—but since meat today is often loaded with hormones, animal drugs and insecticide residues, I'd just as soon leave it alone.

Dr. C. promotes natural foods more than most practitioners. As in any profession there are differences of opinion and some chiropractors are content to advise a more traditional diet, merely suggesting we eat less and cut down on sugar. Others recommend more radical diets of raw foods eaten in special combinations with dozens of vitamin supplements.

The nutritional expertise of chiropractors varies greatly. The bulk of training may be limited to what they learned in chiropractic college, although this represents more than a medical doctor receives. It doesn't qualify a chiropractor to be a nutritionist, however. While some may take further courses like Dr. C. and attain a high level of proficiency and skill, others take brief seminars in nutrition and diet therapy that are designed primarily to add a lucrative adjunct to their regular practice. Know your chiropractor's qualifications before you rely on him or her for nutritional guidance and avoid the hit-and-miss approach to nutrition which many so-called experts practice today. If you have a special problem that goes beyond the expertise of a chiropractor, he or she has an obligation to refer you to the appropriate specialist.

The Basic Four

We need to become self-reliant in our choice of foods. Practitioners from many health fields suggest we simply follow the traditional U.S. government guidelines known as The Four Food Groups or "The Basic Four." However, this standard dietary guide for traditional nutritionists since 1956 has come under attack from progressive nutritionists who favor a more contemporary approach reflecting the original recommendations of the Select Committee on Nutrition and Human Needs.

If you were educated in grade school after 1956, chances are the following food groups are familiar to you:

the meat group

the vegetable-fruit group

the milk group

the bread-cereal group

A growing number of nutritionists, medical doctors, chiropractors, naturopaths, and advocates of food reform (especially vegetarians) feel that such a plan places too much emphasis on meat, dairy products, and highly processed food. It does not encourage us to choose a diet that not only supplies adequate nutrients, but is also low in fat, high in dietary fiber, and relatively free of sugar and harmful food additives. The critics add that in view of the high cost of meat and its negative effects on human health, the "Basic Four" should be revised to reflect the original recommendations of the McGovern Committee and to help the consumer buy more nutrition per dollar spent on food.

Toward a Revised "Basic Four"

Nutritionists say there are six essentials which create a sound foundation for a good diet: proteins, fats, carbohydrates, vitamins, minerals, and pure water. Many believe it is difficult to achieve sufficient amounts of all these elements each day, but they can easily be obtained when we have access to a variety of wholesome foods—whole grains, nuts, seeds, legumes (beans, peas, etc.), fresh fruits and vegetables, and low-fat dairy products.

Shortly after the publication of my book *Eating for Life,* I prepared the following revised "Basic Four." It provides a sound foundation for an inexpensive, nutritious dietary program with a wide range of choice. The revised Basic Four is an excellent complement to regular chiropractic care. In addition to providing vital nutriments for a healthy body, it will help you stay free of toxins, which are among the causes of vertebral subluxations. Since each of us has unique dietary needs, the following food group plan is intended as a general guide.

Protein Group

Three servings daily of dried legumes (chickpeas, limas, black beans, kidney beans, etc.), whole, unsalted nuts and seeds, commercially prepared or homemade protein mixtures (soyameat, gluten, nutmeat, cereal-legume-nut combinations), and low-fat dairy products and eggs (used sparingly). Red meat, poultry, and fish are listed as possible alternates. This group supplies protein for growth and maintenance of healthy tissues, B vitamins which aid in digestion and keep our nervous system in top condition, fat for the production of energy, and minerals (especially iron) that are used to build healthy bones, muscles, nerve tissue, blood, and stomach tissue. Plant proteins (especially legumes) provide dietary fiber as well, which is vital for the elimination of toxins in the body.

Vegetable Group

Three or more liberal servings daily of fresh dark green and yellow vegetables, leafy greens, sprouts, and other vegetables, including carrots, onions, and radishes. This group supplies vitamin A for healthy eyes and skin, vitamin B to maintain a healthy nervous system, vitamin C to help prevent colds and to promote general nutrition, cellulose for the efficient elimination of toxins, calcium which is vital for healthy bones, and iron which promotes red blood cell formation and maintains proper metabolism.

Fruit Group

Three or more liberal servings daily of fresh fruits (including tomatoes) and juices (with no sugar added). Give special attention to sources of vitamin A such as apricots and cantaloupes and vitamin C which is in citrus fruits and strawberries. This category provides an abundance of trace minerals, vitamins A and C, and dietary fiber.

Energy/Fiber Group

At least four servings daily of brown rice, whole grain breads and cereals, potatoes, and other starchy vegetables. This category supplies mostly B vitamins, carbohydrates for energy, protein, and dietary fiber.

What would a typical daily menu look like if we based it on the revised Four Food Group Plan?

BREAKFAST	LUNCH	DINNER
Wholegrain Cereal	Beans and Rice	Lentil Burgers
Fruit	Corn Tortillas	Baked Potato
Milk (animal or soy)	Mixed Green Salad	Sprout-Avocado Salad
Juice	Fresh Fruit	Broccoli
Tea	Iced Herb Tea	Apple Pie
		Beverage

With the aid of nutrition and recipe books listed in the recommended reading section at the end of this book, we can easily create an individualized dietary program. Eating for health can also be eating for pleasure. By experimenting with different kinds of foods (there are over 20 varieties of beans alone) and using them in various casseroles, soups, dips, stews, sandwiches, salads, stir-fried dishes, breads, and hearty desserts, we can not only satisfy our body's legitimate need for nourishment but please our palates as well.

An enjoyable nutitious diet reduces the risk of subluxations caused by food toxins and maintains inner harmony through healthy nerves, organs, and tissues. As you will see in the next chapter, exercise also plays a part in your health by building a strong, flexible spine to resist misalignment and protect the free flow of nerve energy.

10

Staying in Shape: Exercise for a Healthy Spine

CHIROPRACTIC TEACHES THAT OVERALL HEALTH is just a measure of the well-being of the spinal column. In addition to correcting misalignments, many chiropractors recommend regular exercise. Any program can increase our strength, stamina, and coordination, but unless it also strengthens the back and neck to reduce the possibility of subluxations, the benefits are limited.

Like healthy intentions and a nutritious diet, a program of exercise, posture development, and proper lifting can promote constructive survival values in our lives and keep us on the road to good health.

EXERCISE: POINTS TO CONSIDER

Every form of exercise provides some benefits, but not all offer the same advantages. Jogging, skiing, football, rugby, wrestling, dance, and the martial arts are excellent body conditioners, but, from a chiropractic point of view, may be too strenuous on joints, ligaments, and the spinal column.

Jogging, for example, reduces tension, improves our ability to deliver oxygen to all parts of the body, increases muscle tone, and improves blood circulation. However, it jars the body, particularly the spine, and can be a cause of vertebral subluxation. Sports like snow skiing, football, and wrestling often lead to strains of the spinal muscles and bruising injuries to the spinal column itself. Chiropractors generally do not discourage their patients from practicing these forms of exercise, but advise that sports equipment should be in good order, overexertion should be avoided, and complete spinal examinations should be received to determine if there are any physical limitations that could make such exercise dangerous. They also recommend an immediate visit after experiencing any mishaps.

For those who enjoy a sport like jogging but suffer from its jarring effects, a growing number of chiropractors recommend a small trampoline-like device made of a strong steel frame to which a resilient mat is attached by heavy springs. The mat on which you run or jog sits about seven inches off the floor. Research by a testing firm in Houston revealed these joggers produce only about 39 percent of the trauma experienced when we run on the floor. You can write to one of the following companies for more information:

THE JUMP 'N' JOGGER

Jump 'n' Jogger International Corp.
230 Central Park South
New York, New York 10019

THE REBOUNDER

Trim Way Corp.
P. O. Box 77113
Seattle, Washington 98133

SKIP JOGGER

Skip-Hellen Enterprises Inc.
11259 Virginia Avenue
Lynnwood, California 90262

Stretch for Spinal Health

Stretching exercises are among the finest body conditioners and are favored by chiropractors for themselves and their patients. When performed with knowledge and care, they are excellent for firming and toning the muscles of the arms, legs, shoulders, neck, and back. They also firm up abdominal muscles which are directly involved in preventing spinal disorders. According to Thomas Pipes and Paul Vodak, authors of *The Pipes Fitness Test and Prescription:* "When your abdominal strength and endurance are poor, the lower intestines, which are contained in a supporting membrane that attaches to the lower spine, protrude outward, causing disruptive stress on the spine. With continued stress, the backbone eventually distorts, pinching various nerves."

The most popular stretching exercises are featured in the ancient practice of Hatha Yoga. Chiropractors recommend yoga because it helps us relax, improves muscle tone, strengthens the abdominal and spinal muscles, and enables the spine to be more flexible and respond better to everyday stress and strain. There are a number of fine courses on Hatha Yoga available in book and record stores. Classes in yoga and other stretching exercises are offered in most communities. If taught by a qualified instructor, the benefits can be great. A chiropractor from Pittsburgh offered the following advice: "Don't overdo it, and don't force the exercises by straining the muscles or by making sudden movements. Your body is made to move gracefully and you don't have to force it into positions that cause pain and discomfort."

Nine Daily Exercises for Spinal Health

Each chiropractor tailors an exercise program to the individual needs of the patient, often drawing the best features from different exercise systems. The following ones were created by a chiropractor and are especially designed to strengthen the muscles of the neck, abdomen, and back. They reduce tension while improving muscle tone and strength, and are intended to minimize the onset of vertebral subluxations and improve the effectiveness of chiropractic adjustments. Perform these as often as you like, although twice a day is considered ideal. Each can be done by itself or as a group, but all nine should be performed in order to obtain maximum benefits.

Before starting any exercise program, speak to your chiropractor about any possible physical limitations you may have. Those offered here should not cause any pain and can be performed by people of all ages. However, if one or more of the exercises cause discomfort, it may indicate a spinal problem.

Neck Exercises

1. *Cervical (Neck) Extension*

In a standing position, slowly nod your head backwards until you feel a firm pressure at the base of the head (as opposed to letting your head drop as far as it will go). Hold this position for a slow count of three. Slowly bring your head to an erect position once more. Repeat five times. Increase the number daily until you can do 20. Like the following exercise, the cervical extension helps strengthen neck muscles and improve their general tone.

2. *Cervical Flexion*

In a standing position, gently nod your head forward on your chest to the count of three. Make sure to avoid any strain

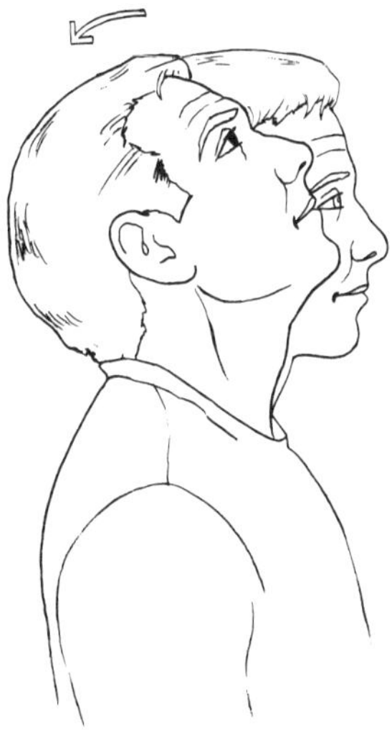

FIGURE 10–1
Cervical Extension

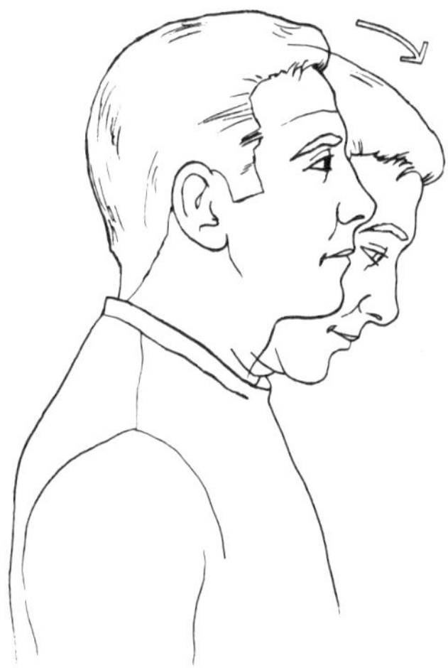

FIGURE 10–2
Cervical Flexion

of the neck muscles. Hold this position for another count of three. Slowly bring your head erect. Repeat five times. Slowly increase daily until you can do 20.

3. *Cervical Left and Right*

In a standing position, turn your head slowly to the left without straining or rolling your head up or down. Hold this position for three seconds. Bring your head back to the center, and rest. Then slowly turn your head to the right, hold, and bring your head back to center once more. Repeat five times. Gradually increase daily until a count of 20 is achieved. The goal of this exercise is to increase the lateral range of motion of the neck and improve muscle tone.

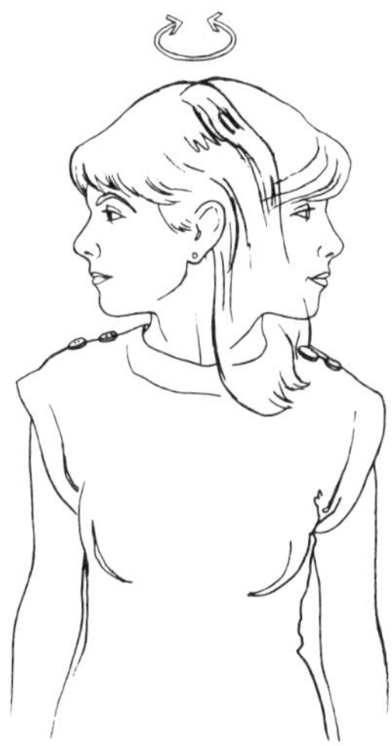

FIGURE 10–3

Cervical Left and Right

4. *Cervical Tilt*

The cervical tilt is designed to strengthen shoulder muscles in addition to those of the neck. First, tilt your head slowly to the left until you feel the muscles on the right side of your neck tighten. Hold this position for three seconds. Bring your head erect again. Repeat by tilting the head gradually to the right until you notice the tightness of the muscles on the left side of the neck. Repeat this right and left tilt three times, and gradually increase daily until you can do 20.

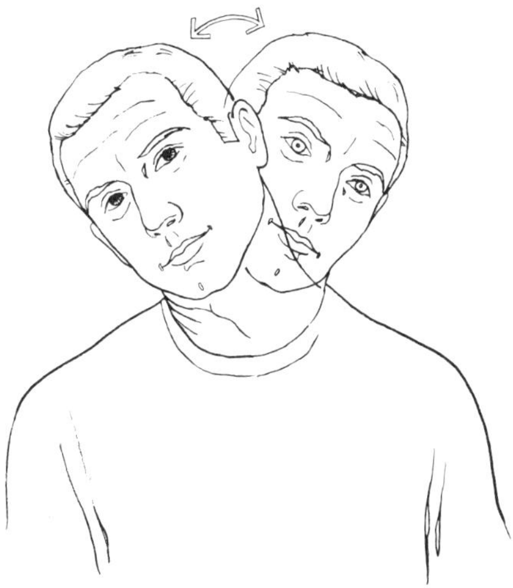

FIGURE 10–4
Cervical Tilt

Exercises for the Mid and Lower Back

5. Thoracic-Lumbar Lateral Flexion

Stand erect with your feet six inches apart and arms at your sides. Slowly lean to the left until your body is angled at approximately 20 degrees or so. You should begin to feel some muscle strain in your right side. Hold this position for five seconds. Slowly stand erect again. Repeat the action by bending slowly to the right. Gradually increase this exercise daily until a count of 20 is achieved. In addition to increasing general body flexibility, this exercise is useful for strengthening the muscles of the middle and lower back.

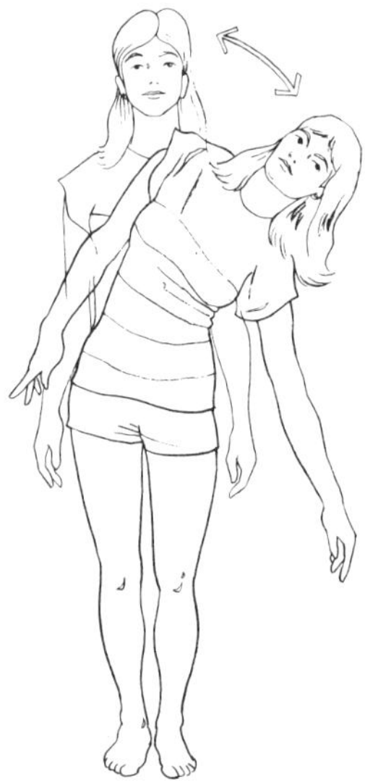

FIGURE 10–5
Thoracic-Lumbar Lateral Flexion

6. Thoracic-Lumbar Flexion

Lie flat on your back. Flex your knees toward your chest—they don't have to touch—and lock your hands around your knees. Gently roll backward and forward letting your head move with the motion; don't try to keep your head flat on the floor. Be sure to lie on a mat, carpet, or other suitable padding, since the flexion will increase the prominence of the vertebrae. Gently roll backward and forward about five times, breathing in when you go backward and out when you roll forward. Gradually increase this number daily until you can do 20. In addition to toning up the muscles of the middle and lower back, this exercise strengthens the abdominal muscles and increases blood circulation.

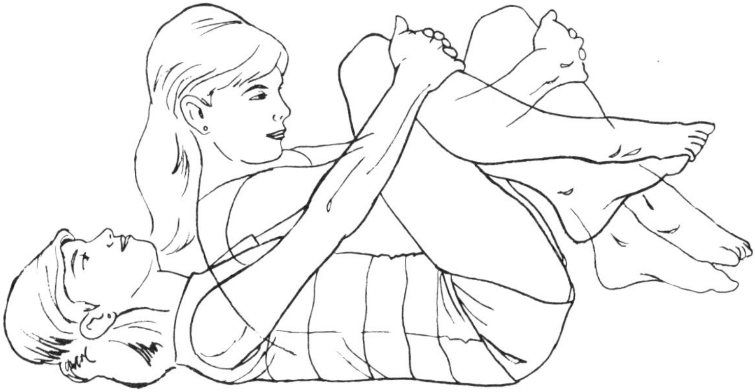

FIGURE 10–6
Thoracic-Lumbar Flexion

7. Thoracic-Lumbar Hyperextension

Lie face down on a carpet or mat with your arms outstretched in front of you. Keeping your arms straight, gently arch your back and slowly raise your arms, head, and shoulders by tightening your back muscles. Raise yourself up, hold for a few seconds, and then lie flat and relaxed. This is a strenuous exercise that will greatly increase the strength of the lower, mid, and upper back, shoulders, neck, and arms. Repeat this exercise five times, and gradually increase daily until you can do 12. (See Figure 10–7.)

8. Thoracic-Lumbar Extension

This is one of my favorite exercises for relieving muscle tension brought about by typing for long periods of time. Kneel down on your hands and knees, with your arms supporting your shoulders. Don't worry about your feet—you can either

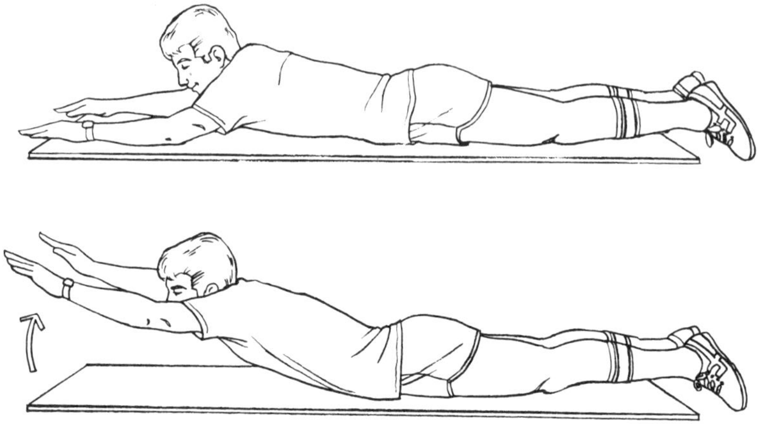

FIGURE 10–7
Thoracic-Lumbar Hyperextension

rest on the backs of your feet or have them lie with the top of the feet touching the ground. Relax your back and slowly slump forward. Hold this position for a second or two and then arch your back to where the spine is "rounded." Roll your pelvis forward when slumping, and backward when arching. This is a good exercise to help you correct some of your own subluxations (you may hear several "cracks" or "pops" as you do the exercise) and tone up the back, abdominal, and shoulder muscles. Repeat this exercise five times, and gradually increase daily until you reach a count of 20.

Exercise for the Abdomen

9. *Abdominal Flexion*

Lie flat on your back with your arms at your sides. Anchor your feet beneath a sofa or a friend. Gently tighten your abdom-

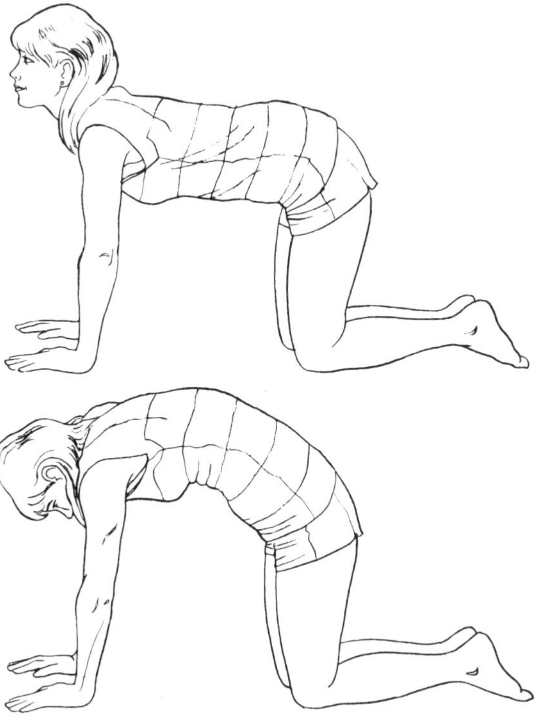

FIGURE 10–8
Thoracic-Lumbar Extension

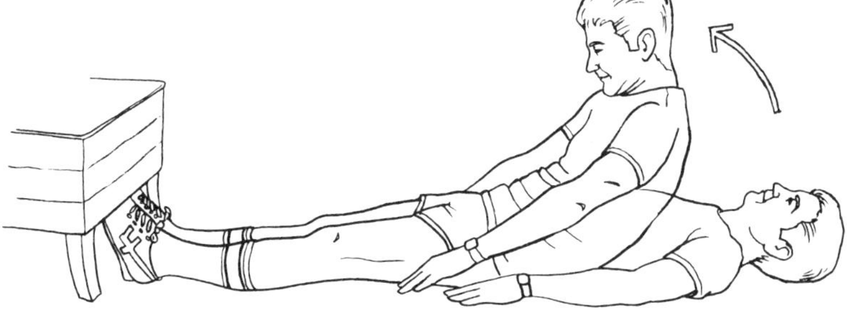

FIGURE 10–9
Abdominal Flexion

inal muscles and raise your body up slowly from your waist, making sure to keep your hips on the floor. Hold for a moment, and then slowly lower yourself again to a position flat on your back. Repeat three times. Gradually increase this count daily until a series of 12 is achieved. This exercise—a variation of the "sit-up"—will strengthen the muscles of the abdomen, upper chest, and legs.

WHAT ABOUT POSTURE?

Good posture is one of the goals of chiropractic. The profession has taken a leadership role in educating parents and children on its benefits for more than fifty years.

Although we were taught that good posture looks attractive and is necessary for coordination, chiropractors point out it also keeps us healthy. When the human structure is out of balance, it can produce distortions of the spine. The resulting curvature may change the position of our internal organs and cramp the lungs, stomach, and intestines which may lead to shallow breathing, faulty digestion, and poor elimination. However, the most serious result is vertebral subluxation which may alter the function of various organs by affecting specific spinal nerves.

There are many reasons for poor posture. Excessive weight, negative emotional attitudes, visual impairment, injury to joints, bones, and ligaments, faulty nutrition, improper sleep support (soft or sagging mattresses), poorly designed chairs, and vertebral subluxations are all common contributors to poor posture. High-heeled shoes, badly-designed seating in cars and trucks, and just plain laziness follow close behind.

Disturbances of body balance may show themselves as a slight tilt of the head to the right or the left, one shoulder (or hip) may be slightly higher than the other, or there may be an abnormal forward curve of the spine (known as lordosis or "swayback") or an abnormal backward curve of the spine (known as kyphosis or "humpback").

Bad posture does not always involve subluxation of the spine, although it usually does. Sometimes spinal curvature may not produce a subluxation and sensitive spinal nerves may not be impaired. However, your chiropractor, as a specialist in spinal care, is qualified to determine the nature and extent of your postural problem. He or she will thoroughly examine your spine, correct vertebral subluxations if needed, and advise how you can develop habits to promote healthy posture.

On Your Feet: Standing and Walking

Human beings are one species of a small group of animals that are bipeds—who stand erect and walk on two legs. This position gives us more agility than other animals, enables us to lift heavy objects, and enjoy greater mobility. It also creates structural demands which can become spinal disorders. For that reason, chiropractors believe learning how to stand and walk properly is essential, reducing the inherent gravitational and structural stress endured every day.

When you stand, point your toes straight ahead. Place your body weight primarily on your heels. Shift your upper chest slightly forward so that it protrudes farther out than the abdomen. Bend your knees slightly. This is not standard military posture, but an easy, relaxed position that reduces forward pull on your back and limits the possibility of strain and subluxation. If you stand for long periods of time, wear low-heeled shoes to reduce muscle strain in the lower back.

When walking, keep the toes pointing straight ahead. Keep your chest uplifted in a natural, unforced way. Be sure to lift your knees so that you are flexing the muscles of the legs and lower back. Wear low-heeled, comfortable shoes with padded soles. They keep your body closer to its natural center of gravity and reduce jarring and fatigue.

At Ease: Sitting and Sleeping

From childhood on, we are told to sit up straight to avoid spinal curvature and other results of poor posture. Although slouching in a chair is a major cause of curvature of the spine, the ideal sitting position is with the shoulders slightly rounded and the knees higher than the hips to prevent back strain and forward curvature of the spine (known as lordosis).

What is the "ideal chair"? According to Hyman Jampol, a physiotherapist who is Director of the Beverly Palms Rehabilitation Hospital in Los Angeles, a good chair fulfills the following three requirements:

1. The seat should be inclined slightly backward for improved lower back support.
2. The back support should be level with your shoulder blades to eliminate stress on the shoulders and neck.
3. Your thighs should be comfortably supported so that sharp edges (like the thin seats of deck chairs) will not cut off blood circulation. If necessary, add pillows to chairs which cause back strain, or cut an inch off the rear legs of a sofa or chair which does not provide adequate low back support. Be sensitive to your body's needs. Learn to avoid chairs and sofas which cause back pain.

Some chiropractors recommend rocking chairs because the backward and forward motion relieves pressure on the spinal muscles and prevents cramping. A small footstool is recommended for keeping the knees higher than the hips. It will take pressure off your lower back and help straighten out the lumbar area of your spine.

All chiropractors agree that a soft, sagging mattress is extremely harmful to the spine. It leads to back pain and vertebral subluxation. Since we spend approximately one-third of our lives in bed, a firm mattress with good back support is an excellent investment in health and comfort.

There are many good beds available in any furniture store. Select one that is really comfortable for you: a mattress that is too soft may allow your back to arch too much. One that is too firm may cause pain and subluxation from too much pressure. A recent survey by the *New York Times* found that most people preferred an "orthopedic" mattress (the King Koil® mattress has received the endorsement of the International Chiropractors Association) with water beds coming in a close second.

The best sleep position is on your back, because sleeping on the stomach arches and strains the lower back and neck. Sleeping on your side is a good idea, especially if you bring both knees up toward the chest to reduce muscle tension in the spine. Conventional pillows often contribute to neck strain, so use a small, soft pillow or special cervical pillow which provides additional support to the neck. Many chiropractors actually sell them although they may also be found in any surgical supply store.

Gezundeit!

A strong sneeze can bring more back injury than almost any other cause. It forces the upper part of the body to bend vigorously. Resisting the sneeze suddenly stops the upper body's natural forward motion, resulting in a powerful muscle contraction that can cause a painful subluxation and lead to an increased lumbar curve. In his book *The Weekend Athlete's Way to a Pain Free Monday*, Hyman Jampol offers the following simple advice: "To prevent injury *bend your knees* so that you are in a half squat and do not resist the sneeze. Relax and let go."

HOW TO LIFT WITHOUT RUINING YOUR BACK

Improper lifting is a leading cause of subluxation. It strains the spinal muscles which can pull one or more vertebrae out of alignment and cause severe pain. We tend to place excessive weight on the lower back instead of the legs which are designed to support far more than our body weight. We lift with a quick, jerking motion and bring about sudden strain. Instead of holding an object close to our bodies, we hold it away from the natural center of gravity, throwing the entire body, especially the spine, out of balance and causing injury and pain.

Learning how to lift properly is not a difficult task. The National Safety Council has recommended the following six steps:

1. Your feet should be approximately twelve inches apart. One should be placed alongside the object you are lifting. The other should be located slightly behind the object. This will provide you with greater balance and stability. You will have greater strength for lifting. If you need to change positions in order to lift, move your feet instead of twisting your body.

2. Keep your back straight in a nearly vertical position. This reduces some of the pressure that builds up in the abdominal region and keeps your spine and body in proper alignment.

3. Keep your chin tucked in. This will reduce injuries to the neck and aids in spinal balance.

4. Grip the object with your whole hand. This prevents it from slipping, which causes a sudden shift in weight and perhaps back strain or other injury.

5. Keep your elbows and arms tucked in. Bring the object as close to your body as possible. With a closer center of

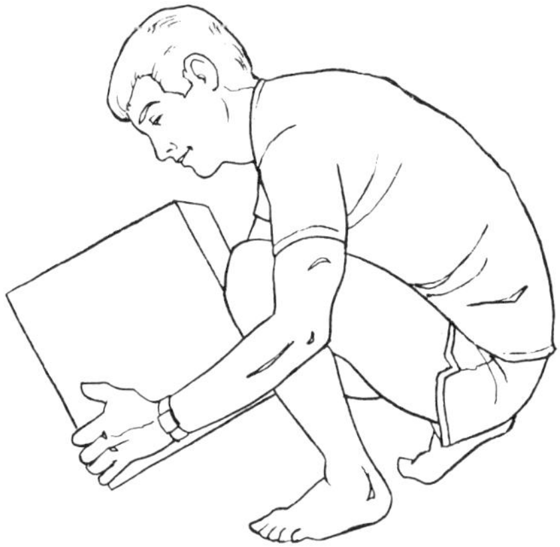

FIGURE 10–10

Feet parted—one alongside, one behind the object you are lifting.

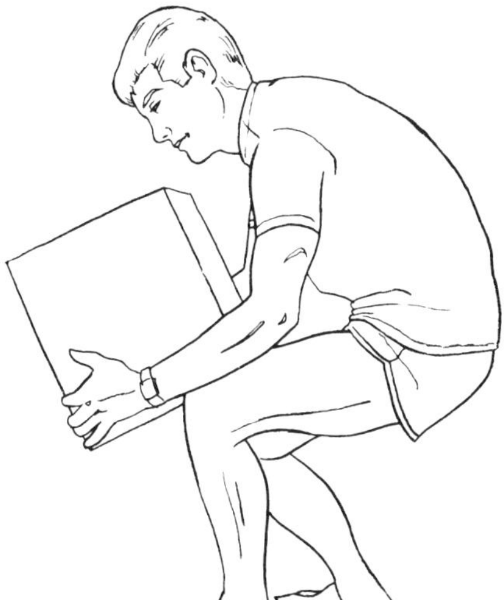

FIGURE 10–11

Keep your back straight, chin tucked in, and grip the object with the whole hand. Keep elbows and arms tucked in.

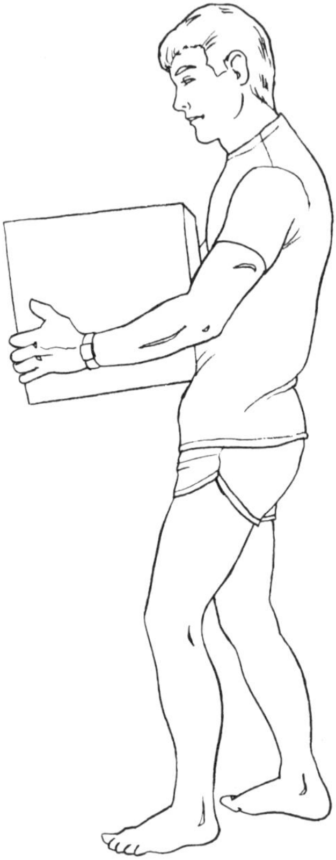

FIGURE 10–12

Make sure that body weight is directly over the feet.

gravity, lifting will be easier and your spine will remain balanced and free from strain.

6. Make sure your body weight is directly over your feet. This will help your body to balance the weight of the object and will give greater strength for lifting and carrying.

WHAT IF YOU SUFFER A BACK INJURY?

The purpose of this chapter is to help you avoid back sprains, strains, and subluxations. However, despite precautions, accidents do happen—a fall in the bathroom, reaching into a low cabinet, a sudden sneeze—which can injure the spine and cause intense pain.

When a back injury occurs, lie down immediately in a comfortable position and apply an ice pack directly to the injured area for ten minutes. Call a chiropractor and arrange to see him or her as soon as possible. Often the cause of back pain, a vertebral subluxation, can be removed with only one adjustment and save you much pain and discomfort. Follow your chiropractor's advice about how you can facilitate recovery.

Through a program of preventive exercise, you can avoid many common spinal problems which cause pain, limit activity, and open the door to ill health. It can even be a pleasure. If you do every exercise described in this chapter, you do not need to devote more than fifteen or twenty minutes a day. Performed to music and in attractive surroundings, daily exercise can be a pleasure looked forward to and shared with family and friends.

Chiropractic works to preserve the integrity of our bodies and keep us healthy, active, and strong. With a personal program of daily exercise and increased awareness of correct posture and proper lifting, you can greatly enhance the benefits of chiropractic care. Take greater responsibility for your health in these and other ways described earlier and work as a partner with your chiropractor to keep healthy.

Epilogue

Chiropractic and Your New Health Future

THE WORLD HEALTH ORGANIZATION DEFINES health as "a state of full physical, psychological and social well-being, not just simply the absence of disease symptoms." Most of us believe good health is our greatest treasure, but according to the United States Public Health Service only three million of us can be termed "healthy" today. According to a recent edition of *The New York Times*, all but 4 percent of our nation's annual health care bill was spent on the treatment of disease. Critics say our present health care system is a disease care system which works on the premise that our natural, physical state is to be sick, and the best way to health is to spend more and more money fighting disease.

The chiropractic alternative teaches that the natural state of human beings is to be healthy. Our body's inborn intelligence is perfectly designed to keep us well and active during our entire lifetime. We have a duty to take responsibility for our health by making sure our bodies function without hindrances of any kind, be they pollution, lack of proper exercise, negative lifestyle habits, or nerve impingement from spinal misalignments.

By taking responsibility for the causes of illness, we become aware of the dynamics of health and how we can make them a concrete reality in our lives. We make a commitment to the prevention of dis-ease rather than focus on crisis medicine. We become self-reliant rather than dependent on a health professional to periodically "fix" our symptoms. This commitment can lead to a new level of self-esteem and a joy in taking better care of ourselves and those we love.

Since its discovery in 1895, the chiropractic alternative has helped millions of people worldwide prevent dis-ease. It has guided them to take charge of their own health. Chiropractic philosophy teaches the body has the ability to heal itself. The chiropractor promotes this integrity by correcting spinal misalignments and teaching patients how to prevent vertebral subluxations through positive lifestyle habits, healthy diets, and proper exercise.

In less than a hundred years, this alternative has become America's second largest health care delivery system. It is chosen by ten million people each year in this country alone. Chiropractic's positive and often dramatic results do not involve the use of drugs or surgery of any kind. Unlike other forms of health care which stimulate or inhibit the body's natural functions, chiropractic's goal is to remove interference to the normal healing process. Chiropractic promotes a respect for the body and its innate intelligence, which distinguishes it from all other forms of health care.

According to a statement attributed to Thomas Edison, "The doctor of the future will give no medicine, but will interest his patients in the care of the human frame, in diet, and in the cause and prevention of disease."

I believe today's chiropractor is the doctor of the future. This preventive care, grounded in a Hippocratic philosophy thousands of years old, will continue to grow because it is safe, effective, and economical. As part of our future, the chiropractic alternative will lead us toward personal responsibility for our health and for the health of our children and grandchildren.

References

CHAPTER 1: THE EVIDENCE: DRAMATIC RESULTS

"Asymptomatic Protruded Lumbar Disc as a Cause of Urinary Retention," *Mayo Clinic Proceedings*, May 1967.

Marcus Bach, *The Chiropractic Story* (Los Angeles: De Vorss & Co., 1968).

The Canadian Family Physician, July 1969, pp. 35–39.

"Cancer and Chiropractic," *International Review of Chiropractic*, September 1977.

E. Celander, A. J. Koenig, D. R. Celander, "Effect of Osteopathic Manipulative Therapy on Autonomic Tone," *Journal of the American Osteopathic Assn.*, May 1968.

"Cervical Vertigo," *The Lancet*, 2, No. 27 (1955).

"Chiropractic Effectiveness with Emotional, Learning, and Behavioral Impairments" *International Review of Chiropractic*, November 1975.

"Changes in the Cervical Spine," *Manuelle Medizine*, 6 (1973).

Chiropractic State of the Art (Des Moines: American Chiropractic Association, October 1979).

"A Controlled Trial of Cervical Manipulation for Migraine," *Australia and New Zealand Journal of Medicine*, 8 (1978).

Commission of Inquiry into Chiropractic, *Chiropractic in New Zealand* (Wellington: Government Printer, 1979).

James Cyriax, *Treatment by Manipulation and Massage* (London: Paul B. Hoeber, Inc., 1979).

D. J. Duffy, *A Study of Wisconsin Industrial Back Injury Cases* (Madison: University of Wisconsin, August 1978).

J. J. Gartland, "Barre Lieou Syndrome," *Foundations of Orthopedics* (Philadelphia: W. B. Saunders Inc., 1965).

"The Good Hands Man," *Sports Illustrated*, July 16, 1979.

K. Gundrum, *Internal Record of Medicine and G. P. Clinics*, January 1956.

J. M. Hoag, "Musculoskeletal Involvement in Chronic Lung Disease," *Journal of the American Osteopathic Assn.*, April 1972.

Journal of the American Medical Assn., 19 April 1971, p. 520.

K. Lewit, *Manual Therapy* (Liepzig: J. A. Barth, 1973).

"Low Back Pain Treated by Manipulation," *British Medical Journal*, 19 March 1955.

Medical Journal of Australia, 14 January 1967, pp. 78–79.

John McM. Mennell, *Back Pain* (Boston: Little Brown, 1960).

"Pathogenic Importance of the Thoracic Portion of the Vertebral Column," *Arch. Orthop. Unfall.-Chir.*, 19, No. 6 (1958).

"Possible Significance of Scoliosis and Asthma," *Annals of Allergy*, March–April 1951.

"Ruptured Intervertebral Discs Simulating Angina," *Journal of the American Medical Assn.*, 15 June 1946.

Herman S. Schwartz, ed., *Mental Health and Chiropractic* (New Hyde Park, N.Y.: Sessions Publishers, 1973).

"Sexual Impotence in Men Having Low Back Syndrome," *Archives of Physical Medicine & Rehabilitation*, November 1966.

Spears Hospital News, May–December 1979 (various issues).

"Spinal Manipulation," *The Canadian Family Physician*, July 1969.

"Spinal Nerve Root Pain Simulating Coronary Occlusion," *American Heart Journal*, January 1948.

"Spondylitis and Hyperthyroidism," *Journal of the American Medical Assn.*, 27 August 1973.

"Symposium: Indications for and Techniques of Spinal Manipulation," *Medical Journal of Australia*, 28 September 1968.

"Syncope, Vertigo, Vision Problems Resulting from Obstruction," *Bulletin of Johns Hopkins Hospital*, 91 (1952).

Time, 19 March 1973, p. 65.

Alexander Towbin, "Latent Spinal Cord and Brain Stem Injury in Newborn Infants," *Developmental Medicine and Child Neurology*, 11 (1969).

Alexander Towbin, "Neonatal CNS Damage," *American Journal of Diseases of Children*, June 1970.

"The Treatment of Subluxation Headaches," *Therapie Genewart*, Heft 5, 1951, pp. 175–179.

Neville T. Ussher, "Spinal Curvatures—Visceral Disturbances in Relation Thereto," *California and Western Medicine*, June 1933.

Chester A. Wilk, *Chiropractic Speaks Out* (Park Ridge, Ill: Wilk Publishing Co., 1976).

M. E. Williamson, "Thyroid Dysfunction and Somatic Reflection," *Journal of the American Osteopathic Assn.*, March 1973.

P. T. Wilson, *The Osteopathic Treatment of Asthma*, July 1946.

A. H. Wolf, "Osteopathic Manipulative Procedure in Disorders of the Eye," *Academy of Applied Osteopathy Yearbook*, 1970.

S. S. Yang, D. P. Corbett, A. J. Brough, K. P. Heidelberger, J. Bernstein, "Upper Cervical Myelopathy in Achondroplasia," *American Journal of Clinical Pathology*, July 1977.

CHAPTER 2: CHIROPRACTIC: A CONTROVERSIAL HISTORY

Francis Adams, trans., *The Genuine Works of Hippocrates*, Vol. 2 (New York: William Wood & Co., 1886).

AMA Principles of Medical Ethics, 1955 ed., Chap. 2, Sec. 1.

"AMA Surrenders to Chiropractors," *New York State Journal of Medicine*, April 1979.

Marcus Bach, *The Chiropractic Story*.

J. H. Breasted, trans., *The Edwin Smith Surgical Papyrus*, Vol. 1 (Chicago: University of Chicago Press, 1930).

"Chiropractic," *University of Toronto Journal of Medicine*, February 1961.

"Chiropractic: Its History and Challenge to Medicine," *The Pharos*, April 1978.

Letter from J. W. Colgan, M.D., to Nicholas W. VanLeeuwen, M.D., August 23, 1963.

Joseph Garland, *The Story of Medicine* (Boston: Houghton Mifflin Co., 1949).

Russel W. Gibbons, *Chiropractic History: Lost, Strayed or Stolen* (Davenport: Palmer College Student Council, January 1976).

Murray Goldstein, ed., *The Research Status of Spinal Manipulative Therapy* (Bethesda, Md.: U.S. Dept. of Health, Education and Welfare, 1975).

Brian Inglis, *The Book of the Back* (New York: Hearst Books, 1978).

F. Le Corre, "Historique des Manipulations Vertébrales," *Les Cahiers du College de Medécine des Hospitaux de Paris*, September 1968.

Letter from D. S. Masland, M.D., to guidance counselors in Pennsylvania High Schools and Colleges, January 23, 1976.

Joseph E. Maynard, *Healing Hands* (Freeport, N.Y.: Jonorm Publishing Co., 1959).

B. J. Palmer, *History in the Making* (Davenport: Chiropractic Fountain Head, 1957).

Daniel David Palmer, *The Science, Art and Philosophy of Chiropractic* (Portland, Oreg.: Portland Printing House Co., 1910).

David D. Palmer, *Three Generations* (Davenport: Palmer College of Chiropractic, 1967).

"Quiet AMA Referral Revision Appears to Affect Chiropractors," *International Review of Chiropractic*, May 1977.

"Radiologists Vow Battle Against Chiropractic, FTC," *American Medical News*, 28 April 1978.

Arthur Scofield, *Chiropractice* (Wellingborough, England: Thorsons Publishers, Ltd., 1968).

"Suit Alleges Broad Conspiracy Intended to Stop Chiropractic," *Hospitals*, 1 August 1979.

Chester A. Wilk, *Chiropractic Speaks Out.*

Memorandum from R. A. Youngerman to H. D. Taylor (Director, Dept. of Investigation, AMA), September 21, 1967.

CHAPTER 3: CHIROPRACTIC: WHAT IT REALLY IS

Brief to the Royal Commission on Health Services (Toronto: Canadian Chiropractic Association, May 1962).

Fu Wei-Kang, *The Story of Chinese Acupuncture and Moxibustion* (Peking: Foreign Language Press, 1975).

Far East Reporter, March 1972, pp. 14–16, 86–104, 106.

Ann Hill, ed., *A Visual Encyclopedia of Unconventional Medicine* (New York: Crown Publishers, 1979).

Brian Inglis, *The Case for Unorthodox Medicine* (New York: G. P. Putnam's Sons, 1965).

ICA Position Statement (Washington, D.C.: International Chiropractors Assn., August 1979).

Journal of the American Medical Association, 26 August 1974, p. 1221.

Eric Martin, ed., *Hazards of Medication* (New York: Lippencott, 1971).

Joseph Maynard, *Healing Hands.*

The New York Times, 25 November 1979, Section 4, p. 7.

Vincent C. Nwuga, *Manipulation of the Spine* (Baltimore: The Williams and Wilkins Co., 1976).

"The Osteopathic School of Medicine," *University of Toronto Medical Journal*, February 1961.

B. J. Palmer, *The Science of Chiropractic*, Vol. 1, 4th ed. (Davenport: Palmer School of Chiropractic, 1920).

B. J. Palmer, *Up from Below the Bottom* (Davenport: Chiropractic Fountain Head, 1950).

Daniel David Palmer, *The Science of Chiropractic*.

R. C. Schafer, *Chiropractic Health Care* (Des Moines: The Foundation for Chiropractic Education and Research, 1978).

Social Security Bulletin, January 1979, p. 5.

Touch for Health Newsletter, August 1979, pp. 1–2.

CHAPTER 4: CHIROPRACTIC: WORKING WITH YOUR NERVOUS SYSTEM AND SPINE

Darald Bolin, *The Philosophy of Chiropractic* (Philadelphia: Dorrance & Co., 1974).

Walter B. Cannon, *The Wisdom of the Body* (New York: W. W. Norton, 1963).

E. Clarke and C. D. O'Malley, *The Human Brain and Spinal Cord* (Berkeley: University of California Press, 1968).

Commission of Inquiry into Chiropractic.

Frank DeGiacomo, *Man's Greatest Gift to Man . . . Chiropractic* (Old Bethpage, N.Y.: LSR Learning Associates, 1978).

Julius Dintenfass, *Chiropractic: A Modern Way to Health* (New York: Pyramid Books, 1973).

FSCO (Lawrence, Kans.: Federation of Straight Chiropractic Organizations, 1979).

Murray Goldstein, *Spinal Manipulative Therapy*.

A. E. Homewood, *The Neurodynamics of the Vertebral Subluxation* (St. Petersburg, Fla.: Valkyrie Press Inc., 1977).

Brian Inglis, *The Book of the Back.*

Donald Law, *The Guide to Alternative Medicine* (New York: Hippocrene Books Inc., 1975).

Daniel David Palmer, *The Science of Chiropractic.*

T. P. Pick and R. Howden, *Gray's Anatomy* (New York: Bounty Books, 1977).

R. C. Schafer, *Chiropractic Health Care.*

Herman Schwartz, *Mental Health.*

Louis Sportelli, *Introduction to Chiropractic*, 4th ed. (Palmerton, Penn.: Louis Sportelli, 1979).

J. P. Warbasse, "Dislocations of Cervical Vertebrae," *American Journal of Surgery*, March 1909.

J. P. Warbasse, *Surgical Treatment*, Vol. 1 (Philadelphia: W. B. Saunders Co., 1920).

Chester A. Wilk, *Chiropractic Speaks.*

CHAPTER 5: THE EDUCATION OF A CHIROPRACTOR

Arturo Castiglioni, *A History of Medicine* (New York: Knopf, 1947).

Chiropractic State of the Art.

Abraham Flexner, *Medical Education in the United States and Canada* (New York: The Carnegie Foundation for the Advancement of Technology, 1910).

Official Directory of Chiropractic and Basic Science Examining Boards with Licensure and Practice Statistics (Glendale, Calif: Federation of Chiropractic Licensing Boards, 1979).

R. C. Schafer, *Chiropractic Health Care.*

Chester A. Wilk, *Chiropractic Speaks Out.*

The official bulletins from all chiropractic colleges.

CHAPTER 6: CHOOSING THE RIGHT CHIROPRACTOR

The Cactus Flower, April 1979, pp. 6–7.

"Chiropractic Comes of Age," *Family Health*, December 1978.

Chiropractic White Paper (Des Moines: American Chiropractic Assn.; Davenport: International Chiropractors Assn.; Cheyenne, Wy.: Council of State Chiropractic Licensing Boards, May 1969).

"Controversy Continued," *The American Chiropractor*, December 1979.

Frank DeGiacomo, *Man's Greatest Gift*.

Samuel Homola, *Bonesetting, Chiropractic and Cultism* (Panama City, Fla.: Critique Books, 1963).

Impulse, June 1979, pp. 2–3, 8–9.

Medical World News, December 11, 1978, pp. 57–72.

B. J. Palmer, *The Science of Chiropractic*.

Daniel David Palmer, *The Science of Chiropractic*.

Pennsylvania Medicine, May 1979, pp. 54–56.

R. C. Schafer, *Chiropractic Health Care*.

"The Straights versus the Chiropractors," *International Review of Chiropractic*, October-December 1979.

Chester A. Wilk, *Chiropractic Speaks Out*.

CHAPTER 7: A VISIT TO A CHIROPRACTOR: WHAT TO EXPECT

"Chiropractors: Healers or Quacks?," *Pennsylvania Medicine*, May 1976.

"Chiropractors Pushing for a Place on the Health Care Team," *Medical World News*, 11 December 1978.

Commission of Inquiry into Chiropractic.

Frank DeGiacomo, *Man's Greatest Gift*.

Samuel Homola, *Bonesetting.*

Journal of Clinical Chiropractic, 2, No. 4 (1968).

R. L. Kane, C. Leymaster, D. Olsen, F. R. Woolley, F. D. Fisher, "Manipulating the Patient: A Comparison of the Effectiveness of Physician and Chiropractic Care," *The Lancet*, 29 June 1974.

CHAPTER 8: HEALTHY INTENTIONS

Herbert Benson, *The Relaxation Response* (New York: Avon Books, 1976).

June Biermann and Barbara Toohey, *The Woman's Holistic Headache Relief Book* (Los Angeles: J. P. Tarcher Inc., 1979).

Norman Cousins, *Anatomy of an Illness* (New York: W. W. Norton, 1979).

Bernard Gunther, *Sense Relaxation* (New York: Collier Books, 1968).

Arthur Kaslow and Richard Miles, *Freedom from Chronic Disease* (Los Angeles: J. P. Tarcher Inc., 1979).

Dolores Krieger, *The Therapeutic Touch* (Englewood Cliffs, N.J.: Prentice-Hall, 1979).

Yogi Ramacharaka, *Science of Breath* (Chicago: Yogi Publication Society, 1905).

H. Saraydarian, *The Science of Meditation* (Agoura, Calif.: The Aquarian Educational Group, 1971).

Hans Selye, *The Stress of Life* (New York: McGraw Hill, 1976).

Hans Selye, *Stress Without Distress* (New York: Signet, 1975).

O. Carl Simonton, Stephanie Matthews-Simonton, and James Creighton, *Getting Well Again* (Los Angeles: J. P. Tarcher Inc., 1978).

Ralph W. Stephenson, *A Chiropractic Textbook* (Davenport: Palmer School of Chiropractic, 1926).

Ernest Wood, *Concentration: An Approach to Meditation* (Wheaton, Ill.: Quest Books, 1968).

CHAPTER 9: EATING FOR LIFE AND SPINE

Nathaniel Altman, *Eating for Life* (Wheaton, Ill.: Quest Books, 1977).

Rudolph Ballentine, *Diet & Nutrition* (Honesdale, Pa.: The Himalayan International Institute, 1978).

E. Cheraskin, W. M. Ringsdorff, J. W. Clark, *Diet and Disease* (New Canaan, Conn.: Keats Publishing Inc., 1976).

"Fat Cats Strike Back," *East West*, November 1977.

George S. McGovern, et al., *Dietary Goals for the United States* (Washington, D.C.: U.S. Govt. Printing Office, 1977).

"Nutrition and Chiropractic," *Bestways*, August 1979.

B. J. Palmer, *Up from Below the Bottom.*

Recommended Dietary Allowances, 9th ed. (Washington, D.C.: National Academy of Sciences, 1980).

Louis Sportelli, *Introduction to Chiropractic.*

Ralph W. Stephenson, *Textbook.*

B. K. Watt and A. L. Merill, *Composition of Foods* (Washington, D.C.: United States Dept. of Agriculture, 1963).

E. D. Wilson, K. H. Fisher, and M. E. Foquay, *Principles of Nutrition* (New York: Wiley, 1975).

CHAPTER 10: STAYING IN SHAPE: EXERCISE FOR A HEALTHY SPINE

Glenn D. Braatz, *Spine Care I & II* (Minneapolis: Spine Care Publishings, 1962, 1976).

Hyman Jampol, *The Weekend Athlete's Way to a Pain-Free Monday* (Los Angeles: J. P. Tarcher Inc., 1978).

Thomas Pipes and Paul Vodak, *The Pipes Fitness Test and Prescription* (Los Angeles: J. P. Tarcher Inc., 1978).

Anne Kent Rush, *The Back Book* (Berkeley and New York: Moon Books/Summit Books, 1979).

Louis Sportelli, *Introduction to Chiropractic.*

Glossary of Chiropractic Terms

The following glossary is intended to offer simple definitions to many terms we encounter which are related to chiropractic.

ADJUSTMENT: The chiropractic procedure of correcting or realigning misplaced vertebrae (*see* SUBLUXATION) in order to reduce nerve interference. Using the bony processes of the vertebra, it is characterized by a dynamic thrust of controlled amplitude. The force and velocity may vary from barely a light touch to a forceful, high velocity thrust.

ANALYSIS: The term used by chiropractors to denote their findings after checking the spine for any nerve interference or pressure due to subluxation.

ANTERIOR: Front.

ATLAS: The first or topmost vertebra of the cervical spine which supports the skull and allows us to nod our heads. The atlas is more subject to misalignment than most of the other vertebrae of the spine.

AUTONOMIC NERVOUS SYSTEM: The part of the nervous system regulating involuntary responses of the body, especially those concerned with digestion, reproduction, elimination, and circulation.

AXIS: The second vertebra of the cervical spine located just below the atlas.

CENTRAL NERVOUS SYSTEM: The part of the nervous system comprised of the brain, the spinal cord, and portions of spinal nerves still encased within the vertebra. It helps the body adapt to its external environment, and involves such processes as sensing and locomotion.

CERVICAL (ser'vi-kal): The neck region which encompasses the first seven vertebrae of the spine.

CHIROPRACTOR (ki'ro-prak-ter): A specially trained health practitioner who adjusts the joints, particularly the spine, mostly by hand with the primary aim of removing nerve interference.

CHIROPRACTIC (ki-ro-prak'tik): "That science which concerns itself with the relationship between structure (primarily the spine) and function (primarily the nervous system) of the human body, as that relationship may affect the restoration and preservation of health." It denotes a system of adjusting misalignments of the spine for the correction of the cause of dis-ease.

COCCYX (kok'siks): A small triangular bone at the lower end of the spine, commonly called the tailbone.

CORRECTION: A term used to denote an adjustment of the spine

CURVATURE: An abnormal curving of the spine.

CURVE: The normal front-to-back curves of the spine as opposed to *curvature*. Maintenance of normal curves should begin during childhood.

DISC: A small pad of cartilage. It is the "shock absorber" located between each vertebra. It provides cushioning and flexibility of the spine and helps to hold the vertebrae in place.

DIS-EASE: Lack of ease or disorder within the body which leads to impairment of bodily health and illness. It is "that condition which allows disease to exist" and is caused by misaligned vertebrae placing pressure on spinal nerves.

DORSAL: A term biologically associated with a region of the spine containing the next twelve vertebrae below the cervical region. This area is also known as the midback or *thoracic* region.

EDUCATED INTELLIGENCE: Denotes acquired knowledge based wholly on training and experience (*see* INNATE INTELLIGENCE).

HIP BONE: Either of the two large bones forming the sides of the pelvis. An imbalance of either of these bones may contribute to subluxation.

IATROGENIC (i-at-ro-jen'ic): Any disease caused by drugs or medical therapy.

ILIUM (il'e-um): The wide, upper crest of the hip bone.

INFERIOR: Below

INNATE INTELLIGENCE: The inborn wisdom of the human body which maintains and coordinates the body functions by way of the nervous system.

INTERVERTEBRAL FORAMEN (in-ter-ver'te-bral fo-ra'men): An opening located between the vertebrae of the spine which provides a passageway for nerves and blood vessels between the spinal cord and the rest of the body. Misalignment of the vertebrae can change the size and shape of this opening causing pressure and irritation to nerves. The primary goal of chiropractic adjustments is to keep this passageway open.

ISCHIUM (is'ke-um): The lower back part of the hip bone; the area upon which we sit.

KYPHOSIS (ky-fo'sis): An abnormal backward curve of the spine. If occurring in the thoracic area, it produces "humpback."

LORDOSIS (lor-do'sis): An abnomal forward curve of the spine. If occurring in the lumbar area, it is called "swayback."

LUMBAR: An area comprising the lower part of the spine located below the thoracic area and above the sacrum. The lumbar area of the spine normally contains five vertebrae. This region is also known as the lower back where subluxations often occur.

MANIPULATION: A generalized manual procedure that resets bones, increases the range of movement, and realigns joint structure in order to stimulate or inhibit body functions.

MENTAL IMPULSE: Impulses which are created in the brain and directed over the entire nervous system to control all cell function.

MISALIGNMENT: A term used to denote a vertebrae out of normal position.

NERVE: A highly sensitive, cordlike fiber which carries impulses between the central nervous system and the body organs and tissues.

NERVE PRESSURE: Abnormal pressure on the nervous system due to one or more bones of the spine being out of place. Pressure on nerves (neurothlipsis) causes loss of normal function and can bring pain, paralysis, and reduced efficiency of a particular organ or tissue.

NERVOUS SYSTEM: The "key" system which controls and coordinates all organs and structures of the human body. It consists of the brain, spinal cord, and a vast network of other nerves which extend to every part of the body. The condition of the nervous system determines to a large degree one's state of health (*see* AUTONOMIC NERVOUS SYSTEM, CENTRAL NERVOUS SYSTEM, PARASYMPATHETIC NERVOUS SYSTEM, and SYMPATHETIC NERVOUS SYSTEM).

NEUROTHLIPSIS (nu-ro-thlip'sis): From the Greek words *neuron:* nerve, and *thlipsis:* pressure. The principle goal of chiropractic is to eliminate neurothlipsis and ensure a continued and uninterrupted flow of normal nerve impulses between the brain and every cell of the body.

PARASYMPATHETIC NERVOUS SYSTEM: That part of the autonomic nervous system whose functions include the constriction of the pupils, dilation of blood vessels, slowing of the heart, increased activity of the glands, and operation of the digestive and reproductive organs.

OCCIPUT (ok'si-put): Also known as the occipital bone, it is situated at the back part and base of the skull, resting on the topmost vertebra of the spine. The spinal cord passes through an opening in the occiput (called the *foramen magnum*) and down through the spinal column.

PAIN: A signal with which the body reacts in self defense to protect its mechanical integrity. Régis, a pupil of Descartes, wrote: "The great engineer of the universe has made man as perfectly as he could make him, and could not have invented a better device for his maintenance than to provide him with a sense of pain."

POSTERIOR: Back (as opposed to front)

SACRUM (say'krum): A triangular shaped bone which forms part of the base of the spine. Originally composed of five segments, it fuses into one bone during early childhood.

SCOLIOSIS (sko-li-o'sis): A lateral or sideways curvature of the spine.

SPINAL CORD: The main cable of nerves within the spinal column extending downwards from the brain. The spinal nerves branch out from the spinal cord and unite the brain with all body organs and tissues.

SPINAL COLUMN: The main supporting structure of the human body, consisting of 24 vertebrae as well as the sacrum and coccyx.

SPINOUUS PROCESS: This is the part of each vertebra which we can see and feel protruding along the back. It is often used by a chiropractor to determine misalignment.

SPUR: An abnormal bony projection from a vertebra or other bone.

SUBLUXATION (sub-luk-sa'shun): A condition in which one or more vertebra are out of alignment to such an extent that a nerve is impinged and the normal transmission of nerve energy is obstructed. The main goal of a chiropractor is to correct subluxations.

SUPERIOR: Above

SYMPATHETIC NERVOUS SYSTEM: That part of the autonomic nervous system made of two cords on either side of the spinal column which is connected by nerve fibers to blood vessels, glands, and muscles. It works opposite the parasympathetic nervous system and accelerates the heart, decreases activity of the glands, etc.

THORACIC (tho-ras'ik): Also known as *dorsal,* it is a term used to describe each of the twelve vertebrae located between the neck (cervical area) and the small of the back (lumbar area).

TRANSVERSE PROCESS: A projection on each side of the vertebra for the attachment of muscles and ligaments.

VERTEBRA (ver'te-brah): A single segment or bone of the spine.

Recommended Reading

HEALTHY INTENTIONS AND STRESS MANAGEMENT

The Relaxation Response. By Herbert Benson, M.D. New York: Avon, 1972.
Simple meditative techniques to manage anxiety and stress.

Guide to Yoga Meditation. By Richard Hittleman. New York: Bantam, 1969.
An excellent beginner's guide to meditation.

Getting Well Again. By O. Carl Simonton, M.D., Stephanie Matthews-Simonton, and James Creighton. Los Angeles: J. P. Tarcher Inc., 1978.
A book primarily for cancer patients, but an excellent guide toward reclaiming and keeping our health. A very important book.

Concentration: An Approach to Meditation. By Ernest Wood. Wheaton, Ill.: Quest, 1968.
A respected classic on mind control and meditation.

Stress Without Distress. By Hans Selye, M.D. New York: Signet, 1975.
How to make stress work for you.

DIET AND NUTRITION

Nathaniel Altman's Vegetarian Book. By Nathaniel Altman. New Canaan, Conn.: Keats Publishing (in press).
Everything you wanted to know about vegetarianism. Includes recipes.

Are You Confused? By Paavo Airola. Phoenix: Health Plus Publishers, 1970.
Clear answers to your questions about vitamins, fasting, raw foods, and more.

Diet & Nutrition. By Rudolph Ballantine, M.D. Honesdale, Pa.: The Himalayan International Institute, 1978.
The finest and most complete book on holistic nutrition available today.

Laurel's Kitchen. By Laurel Robertson, Carol Flinders, and Bronwen Godfrey. New York: Bantam, 1976.
An outstanding guide to healthy vegetarian eating. Includes hundreds of recipes.

COOKBOOKS

Tassajara Cooking. By Edward Espe Brown. Boulder, Colo.: Shambhala, 1973.
Excellent vegetarian cookbook using simple foods.

Ten Talents. By Frank J. Hurd, D.C., and Rosalie Hurd. Chisholm, Minn.: Published by the authors, 1968.
The classic handbook for healthy eating.

Love Your Body. By Viktoras Kulvinskas. Wethersfield, Conn.: O'Mango Press, 1972.
All about raw food and sprouts.

Cooking for Life. By Michel Abehsera. New York: Avon, 1970.
A complete macrobiotic cookbook.

The Moosewood Cookbook. By Mollie Katzen. Berkeley: Ten Speed Press, 1977.
Excellent gourmet recipes from a vegetarian restaurant.

Light Eating for Survival. By Marcia Acciardo. Wethersfield, Conn.: O'Mango Press, 1978.
Four hundred and fifty healthy raw food recipes. A beautiful book.

EXERCISE FOR A HEALTHY SPINE

Yoga 28-Day Exercise Plan. By Richard Hittleman. New York: Workman Publishing, 1969.
An outstanding guide written by a Westerner.

The Complete Illustrated Book of Yoga. By Swami Vishnudevananda. New York: Pocket Books, 1972.
A complete yoga book for the beginner or advanced student.

Integral Hatha Yoga. By Swami Satchidananda. New York: Holt, Rinehart & Winston, 1970.
An easy to follow illustrated guide.

Spine Care (I and II). By Glen Braatz, D.C. Minneapolis (3954 Wooddale Ave., 55416): Spine Care Publishers, 1962, 1976.
Two booklets packed with information about exercise, posture, and lifting.

Bikram's Beginning Yoga Class. By Bikram Choudhury with Bonnie Jones Reynolds. Los Angeles: J. P. Tarcher Inc., 1978.
An excellent yoga book written with humor and charm.

The Weekend Athlete's Way to a Pain-Free Monday. By Hyman Jampol, M.A., R.P.T. Los Angeles: J. P. Tarcher Inc., 1978.
Everything you want to know about stretching.

Index